Renin-Angiotensin-Aldosterone System - Latest Trends

Edited by Takaaki Senbonmatsu and Makoto Katoh

Published in London, United Kingdom

Renin-Angiotensin-Aldosterone System - Latest Trends
http://dx.doi.org/10.5772/intechopen.1003465
Edited by Takaaki Senbonmatsu and Makoto Katoh

Contributors
Aman Singh, Gilson de Abreu Viza Junior, Hao Liu, Hong Zhe Zhang, Krishna Singh, Lana Kourieh, Li Jun Li, Ming Chuan Ba, Ola Arab, Simone König, Vivien Osterhus, Xiao Min Li, Yan Qing Gong, Zi Ce Su

First published in London, United Kingdom, 2025 by IntechOpen
IntechOpen is the global imprint of INTECHOPEN LIMITED, registered in England and Wales, registration number: 11086078, 167-169 Great Portland Street, London, W1W 5PF, United Kingdom

For EU product safety concerns: IN TECH d.o.o., Prolaz Marije Krucifikse Kozulić 3, 51000 Rijeka, Croatia, info@intechopen.com or visit our website at intechopen.com.

British Library Cataloguing-in-Publication Data
A catalogue record for this book is available from the British Library

Renin-Angiotensin-Aldosterone System - Latest Trends
Edited by Takaaki Senbonmatsu and Makoto Katoh
p. cm.
Print ISBN 978-0-85466-873-1
Online ISBN 978-0-85466-872-4
eBook (PDF) ISBN 978-0-85466-967-7

If disposing of this product, please recycle the paper responsibly.

Meet the editors

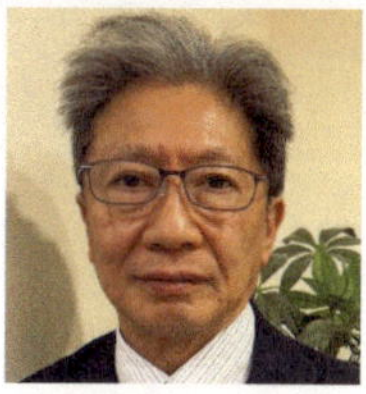

Takaaki Senbonmatsu graduated from Saitama Medical University with an MD, summa cum laude, in 1987. From 1987 to 1989, he completed his internal medicine residency at Saitama Medical Center, Saitama Medical University. After finishing his residency, he joined the Department of Cardiology at Saitama Medical Center, Saitama Medical University, as an assistant professor, a position he held until 1994. In 1994, he moved to the National Institute for Physiological Sciences as a basic science researcher, where he worked until 1996. He focused on protein biochemistry during this time, particularly researching small G proteins. He then moved to Osaka University, where he earned his Ph.D. in medicine in 1997. In 1997, he joined the Department of Biochemistry at Vanderbilt University as a postdoctoral fellow, engaging in research on the renin-angiotensin system. He continued to support the laboratory, becoming a Research Instructor in 2000, a Research Assistant Professor in 2001, and a Research Associate Professor in 2004. In 2006, he returned to Japan as an Associate Professor in the Department of Pharmacology at Saitama Medical University, where he focused on research into (pro)renin receptors and iPS cells. Since 2015, he has been a Professor at the Research Administration Center and the Department of Cardiology at the International Medical Center of Saitama Medical University. He is currently both the Professor and Director at the Research Administration Center of Saitama Medical University and the Department of Cardiology at the International Medical Center. This year, he was also appointed Representative Director of the Metropolitan Academic Research Consortium. Takaaki Senbonmatsu specializes in renin-angiotensin system, heart failure, cardiac regeneration, iPS cells and aging society.

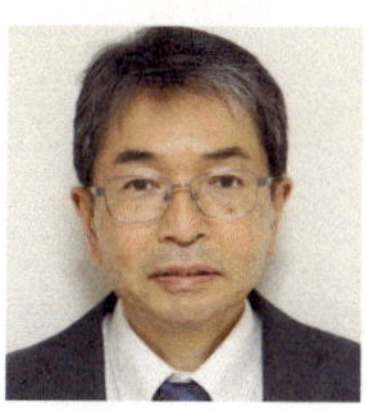

Dr. Makoto Katoh is a researcher specializing in type 2 diabetes, diabetic nephropathy, and cardiovascular diseases. He conducted cardiovascular research at Kyushu University's Department of Cardiovascular Medicine in 1996. He obtained his Ph.D. in Pharmaceutical Sciences from Tohoku University in 1999. With extensive experience in academia and the pharmaceutical industry, he has significantly contributed to retrospective and prospective clinical studies on diabetes and diabetic nephropathy. He has published numerous peer-reviewed articles and currently serves as a Principal Researcher at Naka Kinen Clinic and an Associate Professor at the Research Administration Center at the Saitama Medical University. His expertise includes pharmacology, clinical research, and academic-industrial collaboration, advancing translational research and innovation in diabetes and cardiovascular disease treatment.

Contents

Preface

My encounter with the renin-angiotensin-aldosterone system (RAAS) began in 1997 when I started researching the angiotensin II type 2 (AT2) receptor at Vanderbilt University in the United States. At that time, angiotensin-converting enzyme inhibitors (ACEi) and angiotensin II type 1 receptor blockers (ARBs) were beginning to be used clinically. Many basic research findings demonstrated their effectiveness in treating heart failure—now classified as heart failure with reduced ejection fraction (HFrEF)—and hypertension. Numerous clinical trials were conducted throughout the 21st century, forming the foundation of modern chronic heart failure and hypertension treatment. In a sense, I began my RAAS research at an opportune time. The field was thriving with research on ACEi and ARBs, and as a result, significant progress was made in understanding the angiotensin II type 1 (AT1) receptor and its clinical applications. However, the AT2 receptor, which I was studying, remained enigmatic and highly complex.

At the time, published studies suggested that the AT1 receptor played a pathological role ("heel") while the AT2 receptor had protective effects ("babyface"). It was hypothesized that the best therapeutic approach would involve suppressing the AT1 receptor while stimulating the AT2 receptor. As a result, ARBs were expected to be superior to ACEi in clinical effectiveness. However, no clinical trials confirmed that ARBs were more beneficial than ACEi, and my research did not support the idea that the AT2 receptor functioned as a direct counterbalance to the AT1 receptor. Even today, the role of the AT2 receptor remains unclear.

The history of RAAS dates back to 1898 when Prof. Robert Tigerstedt of the Karolinska Institute in Stockholm, Sweden, discovered renin. He identified a substance with hypertensive effects in rabbit kidney extracts and named it "renin". In 1967, it was confirmed that renin converts angiotensinogen, synthesized and secreted by the liver, into angiotensin I. That same year, it was discovered that angiotensin I is further converted into angiotensin II by angiotensin-converting enzyme (ACE). In the 1980s, the angiotensin II receptor, now known as the AT1 receptor, was identified as a receptor for angiotensin II's physiological effects. The AT1 receptor was successfully cloned in 1984, leading to a detailed understanding of its function and structure as a G-protein-coupled receptor (GPCR). The AT2 receptor was identified in 1993, nearly a decade later.

These discoveries established the classical consensus that RAAS is a crucial systemic regulatory mechanism responsible for blood pressure and fluid balance, acting as a substitute for salt regulation. It was also recognized that an overactive RAAS is a key contributor to hypertension, driving the development of drugs designed to inhibit its activity. 1979 Prof. Miguel A. Ondetti successfully synthesized captopril, the first ACEi. However, the development of non-peptide receptor antagonists lagged behind. The first ARB, losartan, was synthesized in 1986 and approved for use in the United States in 1995. In the 21st century, direct renin inhibitors were introduced, with high expectations for their pharmacological efficacy. However, due to adverse events in clinical trials, their widespread use has been limited.

From the late 20th century onward, researchers have derived common principles from basic and clinical studies, forming a consensus that has shaped current cardiovascular treatment guidelines. These guidelines, established by major academic societies, continue to guide advancements in cardiovascular medicine, with RAAS at the center of this framework.

Over time, RAAS research has expanded. Discoveries such as the prorenin receptor, the existence of tissue-specific RAAS, and the identification of downstream pathways beyond angiotensin II have broadened the field. However, researchers generally agree that the AT1 receptor remains central to disease pathology and a key target for treatment.

Renin-Angiotensin-Aldosterone System – Latest Trends presents 5 chapters related to RAAS:

Chapter 1 "Pathology of the Renin-Angiotensin-Aldosterone System"

Chapter 2 "The Renin-Angiotensin-Aldosterone System: Mechanisms, Pathophysiological Impacts, and Emerging Therapeutic Strategies"

Chapter 3 "Overview of Renin, Prorenin, and the Role of (Pro)Renin Receptor across the Organs and Potential Therapeutic Target"

Chapter 4 "Angiotensin-Converting Enzyme and Blood Basic Carboxypeptidases CPB2 and CPN Activity is an Indicator for Serum Quality: A Quick Lab Test"

Chapter 5 "Subclinical Hypercortisolism"

I have invited many RAAS researchers to contribute to this book, providing a comprehensive overview of the current state of RAAS research. I extend my gratitude to all the authors involved in this work and I hope this book will serve as a valuable guide for future basic and clinical research on RAAS.

Takaaki Senbonmatsu, MD., PhD
Saitama Medical University,
Director of Research Administration Center,
Professor of Department of Cardiology,
Representative Director of Metropolitan Academic Research Consortium,
Saitama, Japan

Makoto Katoh
Research Administration Center,
Saitama Medical University,
Saitama, Japan

Chapter 1

Pathology of the Renin-Angiotensin-Aldosterone System

Aman Singh and Krishna Singh

Abstract

The proposed chapter will involve role of different mechanisms in renin-angiotensin system (RAS) leads to regulation of blood pressure and diseases such as hypertension, heart failure and renal disease. We will also discuss how RAS provides potentials therapeutic target in the treatment of hypertension, kidney disease, and heart disease. There are many drugs which affects different mechanisms of the RAS system and accordingly being used to block different targets in different diseases. We will talk about the success and failures of these drugs. At the end we will discuss clinical trials and their outcomes and how an adverse outcome can be modulated.

Keywords: renin-angiotensin-aldosterone system, blood pressure regulation, angiotensin II, hypertension, heart failure, kidney disease, diabetes, atherosclerosis

1. Introduction

The Renin-Angiotensin-Aldosterone System (RAAS) is crucial for regulating physiology of blood pressure, fluid balance, electrolyte levels and for pathophysiology of hypertension in the body [1]. It involves a cascade of enzymatic reactions and hormone releases that begin with the secretion of renin from the kidneys. Renin acts on a protein called angiotensinogen to produce angiotensin I, which is then converted to angiotensin II by the enzyme called Angiotensin-converting enzyme (ACE). Ang II is a potent vasoconstrictor, meaning it narrows blood vessels, thereby increasing blood pressure. Additionally, it stimulates the release of aldosterone from the adrenal glands, which enhances sodium and water retention in the kidneys, further elevating blood volume and pressure. Overall, the RAAS plays a pivotal role in maintaining cardiovascular homeostasis and ensuring adequate organ perfusion, with dysregulation contributing to conditions such as Hypertension, chronic kidney disease and cardiovascular diseases (e.g. Heart Failure) [2].

2. Renin-angiotensin-aldosterone system (RAAS)

RAAS encompasses a complex interplay of molecules crucial for regulating BP and electrolyte balance. Its activation begins with the release of a renin, stored in juxtaglomerular cells located in the walls of blood called afferent arterioles in the kidneys. This release is triggered in response to several stimuli, such as (i) changes in renal perfusion pressure, (ii) sodium depletion in the body, (iii) activation of the sympathetic nervous system via beta-1 adrenergic receptors - enhancing renin secretion as part of the body's response to stress or physiological demand, and (iv) negative feedback mediated by Ang II, marking the initial and rate-limiting step of the cascade [2, 3]. Renin, an aspartyl protease, is initially synthesized as the proenzyme prorenin, which undergoes proteolytic removal of 43 amino acids from its N-terminus to form mature renin (339–343 amino acids). Additionally, prorenin can bind to the prorenin receptor (PRR), which not only facilitates its activation but also initiates intracellular signaling pathways that contribute to tissue remodeling and inflammation, further linking it to the pathophysiology of RAAS. While renin primarily functioning in the kidneys with a well-known mechanism, it is also found in various tissues including the brain, adrenal gland, heart, and vascular tissues; however, its regulatory mechanisms in these sites are poorly understood [1]. Renin has a unique specificity for its substrate angiotensin (Ang), and it cleaves angiotensinogen (AGT), a precursor protein produced mainly by the liver and released into the bloodstream. Liver continuously produces AGT, to keep a stable level of AGT in the blood. However, AGT transcript is also present in numerous tissues beyond the liver. These include the kidney, brain, heart, blood vessels, adrenal glands, ovaries, placenta, and fat tissue. Several factors can influence the production of AGT in these tissues. Hormones such as glucocorticoids (like cortisol), estrogens, interleukin-1 (IL-1), and tumor necrosis factor (TNF) can upregulate AGT production (**Figure 1**). This occurs in tissues outside the liver, which affects AGT levels in the bloodstream. This process influences BP and fluid balance by contributing to the production of angiotensin II (Ang II), which constricts blood vessels and raises BP. AGT is cleaved by renin to produce Ang I, a decapeptide [Ang (I-X)] which circulates in an inactive form in the blood stream until it encounters angiotensin-converting enzyme (ACE), a dipeptidyl carboxypeptidase, primarily located in the lungs and endothelial cells (ECs) of blood vessels [4]. Ang I is converted by ACE2 to Ang (I-IX), which can then be further converted to Ang (I-VII). These peptides are part of the RAAS, where Ang (I-VII) contributes to vasodilation and BP regulation through its action on the Mas receptor, counteracting the effects of the vasoconstrictor Ang II, which is formed from Ang I by ACE [5]. Within a few seconds to minutes after formation of Ang I, ACE splits two amino acids from Ang I and converts it into octapeptide Ang II [Asp-Arg-Val-Tyr-Ile-His-Pro-Phe, Ang (I–VIII)]—a potent vasoconstrictor and the primary active product of RAAS, and key regulator of BP.

Ang II persists in the blood only for 1–2 minutes and further breakdown or undergoes enzymatic action by aminopeptidase A and N resulting in production of Angiotensin III (Ang II–VIII), and Angiotensin IV (Ang III–VIII), respectively [2]. Ang II exerts significant effects on BP, fluid balance, and hormone release via Angiotensin II type 1 receptor (AT1-R) and Angiotensin II type 2 receptor (AT2-R). These specific receptors, AT1-R and AT2-R, which belong to the G protein-coupled receptor family but signal through distinct pathways with potentially opposing effects. AT1 receptor primarily induce vasoconstriction, while AT2 receptors are associated with vasodilation and anti-inflammatory responses. These receptors are widely distributed in tissues such as the kidney, brain, and adrenal gland, with AT1 predominantly expressed in adult cardiovascular tissues and AT2 more prominent during fetal development [6]. Despite its brief half-life (<60 sec), Ang II regulates sodium and potassium levels by promoting sodium reabsorption and potassium excretion in the

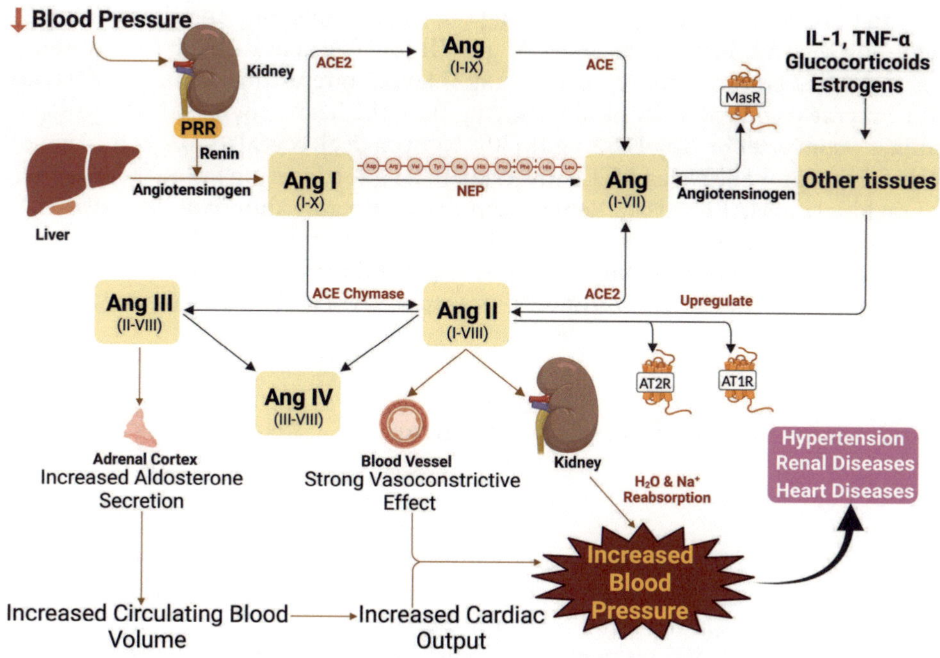

Figure 1.
Overview of the renin-angiotensin-aldosterone system and its role in blood pressure regulation and disease progression. This figure illustrates the cascade initiated by decreased blood pressure, leading to the release of PRR from the kidneys. PRR is converted into active renin, which interacts with AGT produced by the liver to form Ang I. Ang I is subsequently converted to Ang II via ACE. Alternatively, Ang I can be cleaved directly by NEP to form Ang-(I–VII), and through ACE2, to Ang-(I–IX), which is then converted to Ang-(I–VII). Ang-(I–VII) exerts vasodilatory effects by binding to the Mas receptor, contributing to the counter-regulatory mechanisms within the RAAS. In contrast, Ang II primarily interacts with the AT1R, triggering vasoconstriction and enhancing cardiac output. Additionally, Ang II leads to the formation of Ang III, which can then be converted to Ang IV. Ang II also stimulates the release of aldosterone, increasing circulating blood volume and ultimately resulting in elevated cardiac output and blood pressure. The figure illustrates these interconnected pathways, highlighting the complexity of the regulatory system. Conversely, the AT2R is thought to mediate protective effects, such as vasodilation and antiproliferative actions, which can counterbalance the pathological effects of AT1R activation. This coordinated response underscores the dual roles of angiotensin peptides in regulating vascular tone and fluid balance, as well as the potential pathological implications of elevated Ang II levels, which may lead to renal disease, heart failure, and hypertension. The figure also highlights the influence of pro-inflammatory factors such as TNF-alpha, IL-1, estrogen, and glucocorticoids, demonstrating their role in the upregulation of Ang II and the modulation of this complex system. PRR: Prorenin, Ang: Angiotensin, ACE: Angiotensin-Converting Enzyme, NEP: Neprilysin, AGT: Angiotensinogen, RAAS: Renin-Angiotensin-Aldosterone system, AT1R: Angiotensin II type 1 Receptor, AT2R: Angiotensin II type 2 Receptor, TNF-α: Tumor Necrosis Factor-Alpha, IL-1: Interleukin-1.

kidneys, maintaining electrolyte balance and BP. Ang II impacts various physiological processes, including vascular constriction, renal sodium handling, and modulation of brain and nervous system responses to stress, cardiovascular physiology [7–9]. Thus, understanding the RAAS mechanism is pivotal in comprehending hypertension (HTN), renal and other cardiovascular disorders, highlighting its significance in clinical contexts.

2.1 Regulation and significance of angiotensin II synthesis and degradation in physiology

The regulation of Ang II synthesis and breakdown play a pivotal role in shaping its physiological impact. Recently, ACE2, a newly identified carboxypeptidase, has been found to remove one amino acid from Ang I or Ang II, reducing Ang II levels while promoting the vasodilatory effects of Ang I–VII [5]. The delicate balance between ACE and ACE2 is crucial for regulating Ang II levels. Interestingly, while ACE is the main enzyme responsible for producing Ang II, in the heart, chymase is the predominant converter of Ang I to Ang II [10]. Nguyen et al. revealed that activation of the renin receptor enhances AGT conversion to Ang I, triggering mitogen-activated protein kinases (MAPKs) [10]. Renin receptors are notably abundant in cardiac tissue, with detections in the subendothelium of coronary and renal arteries. The tissue-specific effects of heightened Ang II levels and increased RAAS activity hinge on the expression and activation of AT1 receptors, pivotal in cardiovascular and renal pathophysiology.

3. Understanding blood pressure regulation

3.1 The circulatory system

Understanding BP regulation begins with the circulatory system, a complex network of the heart, blood vessels, and associated structures that transport blood throughout the body. Blood is propelled through the circulatory system by the heart's rhythmic contractions, which are coordinated by electrical impulses from specialized cardiac muscle cells. The sinoatrial (SA) node in the right atrium acts as the heart's natural pacemaker, generating signals that cause atrial contraction and blood flow into the ventricles. The atrioventricular (AV) node delays these impulses slightly before sending them to the ventricles, ensuring synchronized contraction and efficient blood ejection into the pulmonary and systemic circulations. Electrical impulses then travel along Purkinje fibers, causing coordinated ventricular contraction and ejection of blood into the pulmonary artery and aorta during systole, which maintains systemic blood flow. Blood from the aorta flows through branching arteries, arterioles, and capillaries, where gas and nutrient exchange occurs. Deoxygenated blood returns through venules and veins to the heart for oxygenation, completing the circulatory cycle (**Figure 2**).

3.2 Blood pressure fluctuation

As the blood flows in systemic circulation, BP fluctuates due to changes in vascular resistance, vessel diameter and distance from the heart. Systolic pressure, the peak pressure exerted during ventricular contraction (systole), is highest in the large arteries near the heart, particularly in the aorta, due to the forceful ejection of blood into the arterial system. As blood moves through smaller arteries, arterioles, and eventually capillaries, resistance to blood flow increases due to the narrowing of vessel lumens and increased friction against vessel walls. Diastolic pressure, the baseline pressure in arteries during ventricular relaxation, reflects the resistance encountered by blood flow in the peripheral circulation. Arterioles or resistance vessels, play a critical role in regulating peripheral resistance and therefore diastolic pressure. Arterioles, controlled by SMCs and influenced by vasoactive substances like Ang II, arteriolar adjust their diameter to regulate peripheral resistance and distribute blood flow according to metabolic demands. When blood pressure decrease, particularly in the renal arteries, the kidney responds by releasing renin, initiating the RAAS cascade. This leads to increased level of Ang II, further enhancing vasoconstriction and

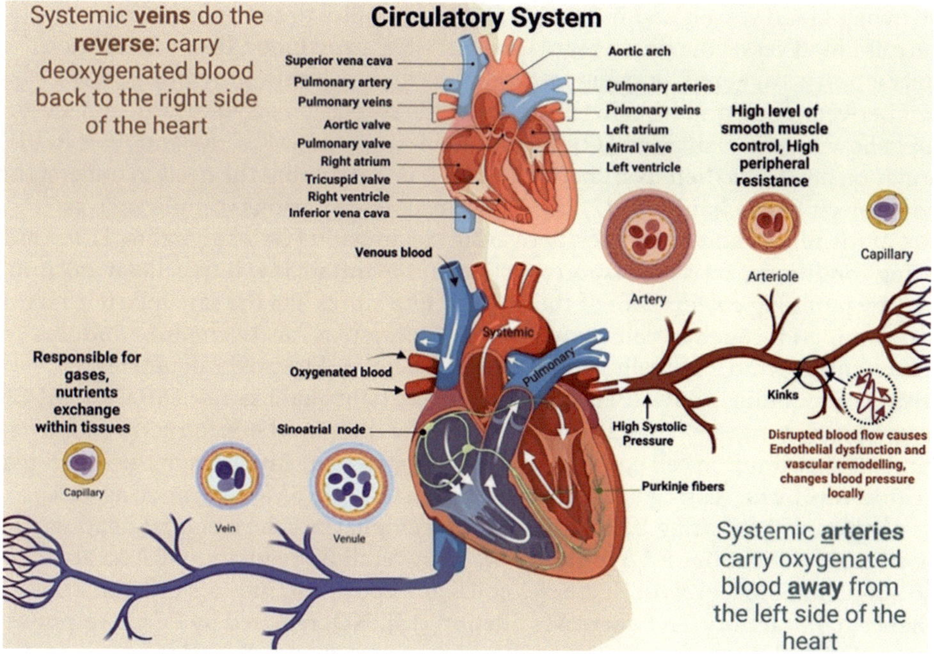

Figure 2.
Overview of cardiac function and hemodynamic changes. This figure illustrates the structural components of the heart, including its valves, and the flow of blood through the circulatory system. It begins with venous blood entering the heart, pumped into the pulmonary artery and systemic arteries, where high systolic blood pressure is indicated. The figure shows arterioles with bends and kinks, highlighting how disrupted blood flow can lead to endothelial dysfunction and vascular remodeling, locally affecting blood pressure. As blood moves to the capillaries, arterioles with dense smooth muscle cells contribute to increased peripheral resistance and blood pressure regulation. Finally, the return pathway of blood is depicted as it moves from the capillaries into the venules and back to the heart, underscoring the interconnectedness of cardiac function and hemodynamic changes.

elevating blood pressure. Throughout the arterial system, blood encounters anatomical features such as bends, curves, and branches, collectively known as "kinks." These features influence blood flow dynamics and pressure gradients. At kinks, blood flow can experience turbulence or changes in velocity, affecting local pressure distribution (**Figure 2**). This over time, chronic exposure to disturbed flow patterns at kinks may contribute to endothelial dysfunction and vascular remodeling, affecting BP.

3.3 Cellular mechanism in blood pressure regulation

BP regulation is a multifaceted process that extends beyond the RAAS. Various cells play pivotal roles in maintaining arterial pressure, ensuring sufficient tissue perfusion in response to physiological needs and environmental fluctuations.

3.3.1 Smooth muscle cells (SMCs)

Smooth muscle cells (SMCs) play a vital role in blood pressure (BP) regulation due to their specialized structure and function. These non-striated, spindle-shaped cells, which range in diameter from 2 to 10 μm and vary in length depending on their vascular location, are primarily found in the walls of blood vessels. By maintaining vascular tone, SMCs directly influence BP [11]. Stimulation causes SMCs to contract, narrowing blood vessels and increasing BP. Their ability to contract and relax finely controls blood vessel diameter, regulating resistance and blood flow distribution. Contraction is triggered by rising intracellular calcium levels, promoting interactions between actin and myosin filaments, while relaxation occurs as calcium levels drop, allowing vessel dilation [12]. Research underscores SMCs' dynamic role in BP regulation and links their dysfunction to HTN, underscoring the need to understand their molecular mechanisms [12, 13]. SMCs respond to various stimuli, such as neurotransmitters and hormones, activating calcium ion (Ca^2+) signaling [12]. Under resting conditions, active transport mechanisms maintain low intracellular calcium levels by pumping calcium out of the cell and into stores like the sarcoplasmic reticulum. Stimulation, such as neurotransmitter binding (e.g., acetylcholine), induces calcium influx from extracellular and internal sources. Elevated calcium levels activate calmodulin, which then activates myosin light chain kinase (MLCK). MLCK phosphorylates myosin light chains, triggering interactions between actin and myosin filaments that result in cell contraction [14]. Importantly, Ang II from the RAAS plays a critical role by increasing intracellular calcium levels in SMCs, promoting vasoconstriction and elevating BP. This interaction emphasizes the essential relationship between SMC function, RAAS activation, and overall BP regulation. RAAS activation also stimulates SMC growth, increases collagen deposition, induces inflammation, enhances contractility, and decreases dilation [15]. NO, released by ECs in response to stimuli like shear stress, enters SMCs and activates guanylate cyclase, converting guanosine triphosphate (GTP) to cyclic guanosine monophosphate (cGMP). cGMP activates protein kinase G (PKG), facilitating muscle relaxation by reducing intracellular calcium and promoting myosin dephosphorylation (**Figure 3**) [16]. This dephosphorylation process allows myosin and actin filaments to disengage, leading to vessel widening and reduced BP.

3.3.2 Endothelial cells

Arteries and veins are structured with sturdy connective tissue and layers of smooth muscle cells (SMCs), lined internally by endothelial cells (ECs), which form a vital barrier between circulating blood and the vessel wall. ECs regulate vascular tone and blood pressure (BP) by synthesizing endothelium-derived relaxing factors (EDRF) [17]. When stimulated by agents like acetylcholine (ACh) or oxidative stress, ECs produce NO, promoting vasodilation and reducing peripheral resistance. The interaction between ECs and RAAS is essential for vascular homeostasis. When BP drops, particularly in the renal arteries, the kidneys release renin, initiating the RAAS cascade and increasing Ang II levels. Ang II causes vasoconstriction and elevates BP, while also stimulating ECs to produce endothelin-1 (ET-1), which counteracts NO's vasodilatory effects [18]. This reciprocal relationship emphasizes the role of ECs in mediating RAAS influence on vascular tone. Additionally, compromised NO production in conditions such as hypertension and atherosclerosis lead to reduced vasorelaxation and elevated BP [19]. Endothelial dysfunction, including endothelial-to-mesenchymal transition, exacerbates conditions like pulmonary arterial hypertension and atherosclerosis, further contributing to elevated mean arterial pressure [20]. Disturbed blood flow patterns, particularly at vascular kinks, induce shear stress that worsens endothelial dysfunction and hypertension. Collectively, these interactions underscore the critical role of ECs in regulating vascular tone and responding to RAAS activation.

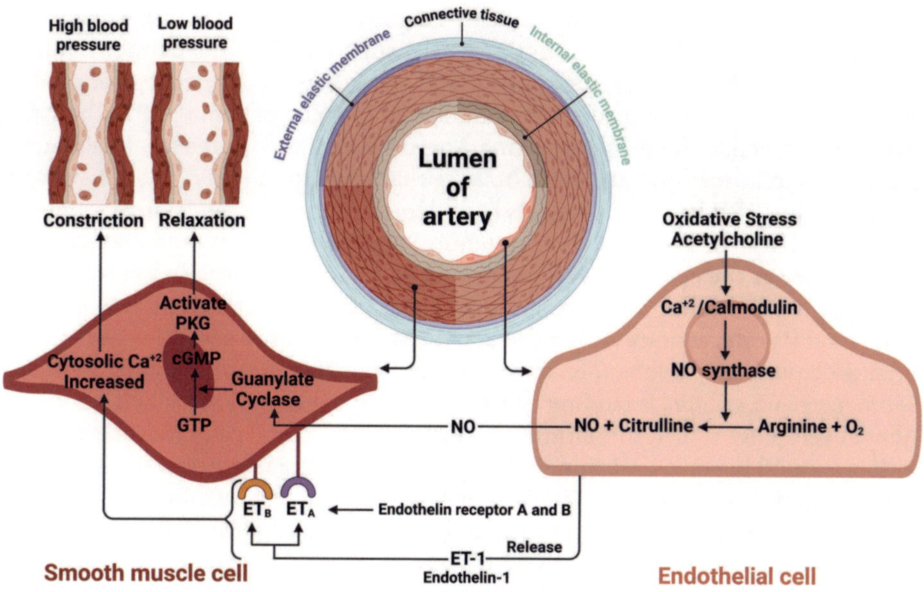

Figure 3.
Endothelial-smooth muscle cell interactions: regulators of vascular tone and blood pressure. Endothelial cells and smooth muscle cells regulating blood pressure. This figure illustrates the structural components of an artery, including the lumen, connective tissue, the inner lining of ECs, and the surrounding SMCs. It begins by depicting the impact of oxidative stress and the neurotransmitter acetylcholine on endothelial function. These factors activate calcium/calmodulin pathways, stimulating NO synthase, which catalyzes the conversion of oxygen and arginine into NO and citrulline. The generated NO diffuses into adjacent SMCs, activating guanylate cyclase. This enzyme facilitates the conversion of GTP to cGMP. The increase in cGMP activates PKG, resulting in smooth muscle relaxation and a subsequent decrease in blood pressure. In parallel, the figure illustrates the release of ET-1 from ECs. ET-1 binds to its receptors, ETA and ETB, located on the SMCs. This interaction triggers an increase in cytosolic calcium levels within the SMC, leading to contraction and an increase in blood pressure. The relationship between ECs and SMCs is critical for regulating vascular tone and blood pressure; endothelial cells produce vasodilators like NO that promote relaxation of SMC, while also releasing vasoconstrictors like ET-1 that induce contraction. This balance is essential for maintaining proper hemodynamics and responding to physiological changes. SMC: Smooth Muscle Cell, NO: Nitric Oxide, ET-1: Endothelin-1, ETA: Endothelin A Receptor, ETB: Endothelin B Receptor, GTP: Guanosine Triphosphate, cGMP: Cyclic Guanosine Monophosphate, PKG: Protein Kinase G.

3.3.3 Renal tubular cells

Renal tubular cells, integral components of the nephron within the kidney, are essential for maintaining BP through complex mechanisms of fluid and electrolyte handling, hormonal regulation, and neural signaling responses. These epithelial cells line the nephron and are organized into distinct segments: proximal tubules, loops of Henle, distal convoluted tubules, and collecting ducts. Among these, juxtaglomerular cells, located in the afferent arterioles, play a critical role by releasing renin in response to decreased renal perfusion pressure or low sodium (Na^+) levels. The ability of renal tubular cells to participate in renal autoregulation is vital for sustaining a constant glomerular filtration rate (GFR) and renal blood flow, even amidst fluctuations in systemic pressure. This autoregulatory capacity helps stabilize BP and ensures efficient kidney function. The prorenin receptor (PRR) pathway in renal tubular cells is pivotal for BP regulation and sodium balance. PRR, a multifunctional protein encoded by the ATP6AP2 gene, is expressed throughout various segments of the renal tubules, particularly in collecting ducts [21]. PRR interacts with both prorenin and renin to catalyze the conversion of AGT into Ang I, which is then transformed into Ang II. Importantly, PRR activates both Ang II-dependent and independent signaling pathways [10]. When prorenin binds to PRR, it enhances the cleavage of AGT, which is essential for Ang II production. Similarly, binding of renin to PRR boosts its catalytic efficiency, further promoting Ang II generation. Moreover, PRR plays a role in sodium reabsorption and fluid balance that is independent of Ang II signaling. Studies utilizing PRR knockout models have demonstrated its crucial involvement in modulating BP dynamics and sodium retention mechanisms. This includes influencing the activity of the epithelial Na^+ channel (ENaC) through protein kinase A (PKA) and Akt pathways, highlighting the importance of PRR in electrolyte homeostasis [22]. Beyond its interactions within the RAAS, PRR engages in several other critical cellular processes. It is involved in autophagy and Wnt/β-catenin signaling with multiple downstream effects, including cell survival and proliferation, which are vital for cellular development, differentiation, and metabolism. These roles indicate that PRR's functions extend beyond traditional BP regulation, linking it to broader physiological and pathophysiological contexts, including hypertension and metabolic syndrome [23]. Despite the established importance of PRR, there is ongoing debate regarding its classification as a traditional factor within the RAAS. While it clearly interacts with components of this system, its diverse functions suggest a more complex role that warrants further investigation.

3.4 RAAS in regulation of blood pressure

Research on Ang II's role in cellular growth shows its impact on BP elevation. For instance, studies in rats have demonstrated that a two-week infusion of Ang II induces HTN and hypertrophy of vascular smooth muscle cells (VSMCs) [24]. Elevated BP also induces shear stress, which in turn upregulates Ang II receptors thereby linking high BP to vascular remodeling [25]. Thus, RAAS plays a crucial role in the regulation of BP through various mechanisms involving vasoconstriction, sodium retention, and aldosterone secretion. This system is pivotal in maintaining homeostasis and responding to changes in blood volume and pressure and Ang II is a key component of the RAAS-exerts its vasoconstrictive effects primarily through binding to AT1 receptors on VSMCs. This interaction triggers intracellular signaling pathways that lead to smooth muscle contraction and subsequent vasoconstriction.

3.4.1 Mechanism of vasoconstriction

Ang II interacts primarily with AT1 receptors concentrated in arteries, arterioles, and veins, triggering intracellular signaling pathways essential for vasoconstriction and BP regulation [26]. Upon binding, Ang II activates G-protein coupled pathways, leading to phospholipase C (PLC) activation [24]. PLC breaks down phosphatidylinositol 4,5-bisphosphate (PIP2) into inositol trisphosphate (IP3) and diacylglycerol (DAG). IP3 releases calcium ions (Ca2+) from intracellular stores, while DAG activates protein kinase C (PKC). PKC enhances contractile protein responsiveness to Ca^{2+}, activating myosin light chain kinase (MLCK), which phosphorylates myosin light chains. This process causes contraction of VSMCs, particularly in arterioles, increasing peripheral vascular resistance and systemic BP [27]. Veins, with larger lumens and less SMCs, exhibit minimal vasoconstrictive response to Ang II, allowing them to accommodate changes in blood volume effectively without significant tone changes [26].

3.4.2 Sodium retention and aldosterone secretion

Sodium retention and aldosterone secretion are crucial for blood pressure (BP) regulation via the RAAS. Angiotensin II (Ang II) stimulates aldosterone release from the adrenal cortex, which is essential for kidney function and fluid balance. Aldosterone binds to mineralocorticoid receptors in the distal convoluted tubules and collecting ducts, triggering the transcription of genes for epithelial sodium channels (ENaC) and sodium-potassium ATPases (Na^+/K^+ ATPase). This increases sodium reabsorption from renal filtrate into the bloodstream, boosting blood volume, cardiac output, and BP [28]. Aldosterone also promotes potassium and hydrogen ion excretion, maintaining electrolyte balance. Additionally, Ang II enhances sodium reabsorption in the proximal tubule and thick ascending limb of the loop of Henle, further elevating BP [29]. Consequently, elevated Ang II levels lead to long-term adjustments in arterial pressure.

3.4.3 Impact of angiotensin II on cell function and blood pressure

Ang II primarily targets VSMCs but also has a profound impact on endothelial cells, contributing to endothelial dysfunction and influencing BP regulation. In ECs, Ang II stimulates the production of ROS, activates apoptotic pathways, and promotes thrombosis. Initially, Ang II enhances NO production by upregulating endothelial nitric oxide synthase (eNOS) mRNA, which supports vascular relaxation [30]. However, elevated Ang II levels induce oxidative stress, impairing endothelial function and contributing to endothelial dysfunction [31]. Intracellular ROS activate nuclear factor κB (NF-κB), leading to increased expression of adhesion molecules like intercellular adhesion molecule-1 (ICAM-1) and vascular cell adhesion molecule-1 (VCAM-1) on ECs. This promotes vascular inflammation and atherosclerosis progression. Ang II also affects the secretion of inflammatory cytokines such as TNF-α, which exacerbates vascular inflammation and is elevated in vascular disorders. This cytokine production is further amplified by Ang II through a PKC-dependent pathway in macrophages [32]. Additionally, Ang II disrupts the balance between thrombosis and fibrinolysis by increasing plasminogen-activator inhibitor type 1 (PAI-1) mRNA levels in both ECs and VSMCs. This inhibition of fibrinolysis, combined with Ang II-induced upregulation of adhesion molecules and the LDL receptor in ECs, further exacerbates atherosclerosis [33]. These mechanisms collectively highlight Ang II's significant role in modulating endothelial function, contributing to endothelial dysfunction and inflammation, and ultimately influencing BP regulation through its effects on vascular tone and integrity. Ang II can both promote and inhibit EC apoptosis, with its effects modulated by factors such as oxidized low-density lipoprotein (oxLDL). Evidence suggests that both AT1 and AT2 receptors are involved in mediating EC apoptosis, with the balance between their expression levels being crucial in determining Ang II's impact on endothelial cells [34].

3.5 Hormonal/physiological regulation of blood pressure

Physical activity significantly influences BP regulation through various physiological mechanisms. The initial study in 1968 revealed that men who exercised more than 5 hrs/week had a lower risk of developing HTN later in life [35]. This finding was further supported by Boyer and Kasch, showed that aerobic exercise reduced BP in men with HTN [36]. BP regulation involves intricate interactions

Hormone/ Peptide	Source	Receptors	Actions	Clinical significance
Aldosterone	Adrenal cortex	*Mineralocorticoid receptor (MR)*	Increases Na^+ reabsorption, K^+ and H^+ excretion	Regulates blood volume and electrolyte balance, contributes to hypertension [40]
Natriuretic Peptides (ANP, BNP)	Atria (ANP), Ventricles (BNP)	*NPR-A (ANP), NPR-B (BNP)*	Inhibit RAAS, regulate fluid/electrolyte balance, decrease sympathetic tone, vasodilation	Used as markers for ventricular hypertrophy and heart failure severity [39]
Vasopressin (ADH)	Hypothalamus	*V1A, V1B, V2*	Increases water permeability in collecting ducts, vasoconstriction	Regulates water balance, responds to changes in plasma osmolality/volume [41]
Substance P	Intestine, CNS	*NK1 receptor*	Vasodilation, pain transmission modulation	Modulates neuroendocrine function, role in vascular tone regulation [42]
Adipokines (Adiponectin, Leptin)	Adipose tissue	*AdipoR1, AdipoR2*	Vasorelaxation, anti-inflammatory effects, metabolic regulation	Protects against endothelial dysfunction, links obesity to BP regulation [43]
Kallikrein-Kinin System	Various tissues	*B1, B2 receptors*	Vasodilation via NO release, BP regulation	Interacts with ACE inhibitors, effect systemic hemodynamics [43]

This table summarizes key hormones and peptides involved in blood pressure regulation, including their production sites, receptors, actions, and clinical relevance. Aldosterone from the adrenal cortex acts on mineralocorticoid receptors to increase sodium reabsorption and excrete potassium and hydrogen ions, contributing to hypertension. Natriuretic peptides (ANP and BNP), secreted from the atria and ventricles, inhibit the RAAS and promote vasodilation, serving as markers for heart conditions. Vasopressin (ADH), produced in the hypothalamus, increases water permeability and induces vasoconstriction, regulating water balance. Substance P, found in the intestine and CNS, promotes vasodilation and modulates pain transmission, impacting vascular tone. Adipokines like adiponectin and leptin from adipose tissue facilitate vasorelaxation and link obesity to blood pressure regulation. The Kallikrein-Kinin system induces vasodilation through nitric oxide release and interacts with ACE inhibitors to affect hemodynamics. ANP: Atrial Natriuretic Peptide, BNP: B-type Natriuretic Peptide, BP: Blood Pressure, RAAS: Renin-Angiotensin-Aldosterone System, CNS: Central Nervous System, NO: Nitric Oxide, MR: Mineralocorticoid Receptor, NPR: Natriuretic Peptide Receptor, V1A/V1B/V2: Vasopressin Receptors, NK1: Neurokinin 1 Receptor, AdipoR1/AdipoR2: Adiponectin Receptors.

Table 1.
Hormones and peptides involved in blood pressure regulation.

between hormonal systems and physiological responses, with physical activity playing a significant role [37]. Regular aerobic exercise, such as running/swimming, initially increases heart rate and cardiac output to meet metabolic demands, temporarily elevating BP. Over time, chronic aerobic exercise leads to adaptations that enhance cardiovascular health and contribute to BP control [38]. Exercise stimulates RAAS, leading to the production of Ang II, temporarily raises BP during physical activity. Regular aerobic exercise enhances the efficiency of this system, thereby improving bp regulation over time. Additionally, physical activity influences the secretion of natriuretic peptides, such as atrial natriuretic peptide (ANP) and brain natriuretic peptide (BNP), which are released from the heart in response to increased cardiac wall tension during exercise. These peptides enhance vasodilation, increase Na + and H2O excretion, and inhibit RAAS activity, collectively contributing to lower bp [39]. **Table 1** provides a comprehensive overview of key hormones and peptides crucial for maintaining BP:

4. Health risk of high blood pressure

High BP, or HTN, poses significant health risks if not properly managed. Persistent elevation in BP strains arteries, increasing the risk of severe cardiovascular conditions such as coronary artery disease, heart attack, and stroke [44]. This continuous pressure can lead to atherosclerosis, where plaque buildup narrows arteries and restricts blood flow, further exacerbating cardiovascular risks [45]. HTN also endangers kidney health, potentially leading to chronic kidney disease (CKD) or failure [46]. Population studies reveal that as systolic blood pressure (SBP) rises, particularly to levels ≥115 mmHg, the incidence of cardiovascular events such as stroke, heart failure, and premature mortality increases [47]. High BP also elevates the risk of vision impairment through retinopathy and raises the likelihood of transient ischemic attacks (TIAs) and strokes, which can cause permanent neurological damage or death [48, 49]. Additionally, HTN contributes to metabolic syndrome—a cluster of conditions including obesity, high blood sugar, abnormal cholesterol levels, and increased abdominal fat—which collectively heighten the risk of diabetes and cardiovascular disease [50–52]. Understanding the role of the RAAS in BP regulation and its complex involvement in HTN, kidney and heart failure is essential for developing effective therapeutic strategies to manage these conditions.

4.1 Hypertension

Hypertension is characterized by persistently elevated BP levels above the normal range, typically indicated by readings such as 120/80 mm Hg [53]. Healthy BP is below 120 mm Hg SBP and 80 mm Hg. HTN is diagnosed with SBP ≥ 130 mm Hg and/or DBP ≥ 80 mm Hg, necessitating monitoring and management to mitigate associated health risks [54]. HTN can result from a variety of factors, involving intricate interactions between genetic predispositions and lifestyle choices. Atherosclerosis, characterized by arterial narrowing and plaque buildup, significantly contributes to HTN by increasing resistance to blood flow [45]. Endothelial dysfunction, characterized by a shift in endothelial cells towards a more mesenchymal phenotype, contributes to vascular calcification and atherosclerosis, further complicating HTN by reducing arterial elasticity and promoting plaque formation [20]. As endothelial cells directly contribute to atherosclerosis and other CVDs disease and its show direct and indirect effect on HTN. Understanding whether endothelial dysfunction precedes HTN or vice versa could provide insights into early diagnostic markers or therapeutic targets. HTN often coexists with obesity, physical inactivity, high salt intake, excessive alcohol consumption, and chronic stress. Additionally, it frequently accompanies conditions such as diabetes mellitus, CKD, and sleep apnea, collectively termed comorbidities. A Canadian study of hypertensive patients aged 35 years and older revealed significant associations with obesity, diabetes, and hyperlipidemia, suggesting shared underlying factors [55]. Understanding these complex interactions is crucial in comprehensively addressing the causes and management of HTN.

4.1.1 Diabetes, RAAS and hypertension

The RAAS in adipose tissue plays critical roles in adipogenesis, lipid and glucose metabolism, and inflammation regulation [56]. In obesity, adipocyte hypertrophy (*enlargement of fat cells*) and cellular hypoxia (*low oxygen level in cells*) lead to increased oxidative stress and inflammation, prompting macrophage infiltration and the release of inflammatory mediators, including Ang II [57]. Elevated Ang II levels are implicated in obesity-related hypertension and insulin resistance [56]. Adipocytes also produce AGT, further stimulating RAAS activity. In diabetes mellitus, hyperglycemia induces oxidative stress and endothelial dysfunction, upregulating Ang II receptors on VSMCs. Heightened Ang II signaling exacerbates vasoconstriction and promotes vascular remodeling, contributing to HTN. Additionally, insulin resistance in diabetes enhances renal sodium reabsorption via increased proximal tubular sodium-hydrogen exchanger activity, exacerbating RAAS-mediated hypertension. Studies on cell cultures reveal adipocytes expressing aldosterone synthase, with elevated aldosterone production in adipocytes from db/db mice, a model of diabetes-associated obesity. Inhibiting aldosterone with eplerenone in this model improves arterial endothelial dysfunction, indicating adipocyte-derived aldosterone's role in vascular stiffness and resistant hypertension [58].

4.1.2 Atherosclerosis, RAAS and hypertension

Atherosclerosis, a chronic inflammatory disease of the arteries, significantly influences RAAS activity, contributing to the pathogenesis of HTN through intricate mechanisms: (i) *Endothelial Dysfunction*: Atherosclerosis initiates with endothelial dysfunction, marked by diminished NO availability and increased expression of adhesion molecules, including VCAM-1 and ICAM-1. These alterations promote leukocyte adhesion and infiltration into the vascular wall, triggering local inflammation [59]. Ang II activates NF-κB in endothelial cells and other cell types, leading to the production of monocyte chemoattractant protein-1 (MCP-1), cytokines such as IL-6, IL-8, and TNF-α [60, 61]. Consequently, endothelial cells upregulate AT1Rs at sites of vessel wall injury, enhancing Ang II responsiveness [62]. Ang II then stimulates vasoconstriction, boosts aldosterone secretion, and promotes sodium reabsorption, collectively contributing to elevated BP. (ii) *Oxidative Stress* and *Ang II Production*: Oxidative stress, a hallmark of atherosclerosis, increases Ang II production within the arterial wall. ROS generated by activated macrophages and ECs stimulate AGT synthesis in VSMCs. Ang II then acts locally to promote SMCs proliferation and vascular remodeling. In VSMCs, Ang II induces the production of MCP-1 and IL-6 through NAD(P)H oxidase activation [63, 64]. This inflammatory milieu is further compounded by elevated levels of other inflammatory cytokines, such as IL-18, which are prominent in human atherosclerotic plaques. Ang II enhances the effects of IL-18 by activating NF-κB and promoting STAT 3-mediated expression of IL-18α receptors, thereby, exacerbates vascular hypertrophy, narrowing arterial lumens and increasing systemic vascular resistance, which contributes to HTN. (iii). *Plaque Formation and Systemic RAAS Activation*: Advanced atherosclerosis leads to plaque formation, characterized by lipid accumulation, fibrosis, and calcification within arterial walls. Plaque rupture or erosion exposes thrombogenic materials to the bloodstream, triggering platelet activation and thrombus formation. Ischemic tissue injury and increased sympathetic nervous system activity due to atherosclerotic plaque instability result in systemic RAAS activation [65]. Elevated plasma Ang II levels further enhance vasoconstriction, sodium retention, and aldosterone-mediated volume expansion, exacerbating HTN. Ang II infusion in apolipoprotein E-deficient mice accelerates atherosclerosis and aneurysm formation demonstrating the role of Ang II in advancing these processes [24].

4.1.3 Treatment options

According to the World Health Organization, approximately 1.28 billion adults aged 30–79 have HTN [66]. Effective management is essential to achieve normal BP and reduce associated risks. Treatment typically involves a combination of antihypertensive medications targeting key physiological pathways. Angiotensin-converting enzyme inhibitors (ACEis) such as enalapril and lisinopril, block the conversion of Ang I to Ang II, a potent vasoconstrictor. Angiotensin receptor blockers (ARBs), such as losartan and valsartan, prevent Ang II from binding to its receptors, thus promoting vasodilation and lowering BP [52]. Calcium channel blockers (CCBs), including amlodipine and diltiazem, inhibit calcium entry into arterial and cardiac smooth muscle cells, aiding vasodilation and improving myocardial oxygen supply, particularly in coronary artery disease [67]. Thiazide diuretics, like indapamide and chlorthalidone, increase sodium and water excretion by the kidneys, reducing blood volume and effectively lowering BP, making them a preferred first-line therapy due to their efficacy in reducing cardiovascular morbidity and mortality [68].

4.1.4 Current and emerging RAAS-targeted therapies for hypertension: Clinical efficacy and safety

Medications targeting the RAAS, such as ACE inhibitors and ARBs, manage hypertension by blocking Ang II production or its effects on blood vessels. RAAS antagonists and certain dihydropyridine CCBs enhance NO bioavailability, reduce oxidative stress, and suppress inflammation, thereby improving endothelial function and vascular health [69, 70]. Aldosterone antagonists, such as spironolactone, block aldosterone at its receptors and are critical in treating resistant hypertension, which remains high despite the use of three antihypertensive agents, including a diuretic [71]. Primary aldosteronism (*a condition characterized by excessive production of aldosterone from the adrenal glands, leading to hypertension and electrolyte imbalances*) and mild hyperaldosteronism (*a less severe form of aldosteronism with slightly elevated levels of aldosterone*) often contribute to this condition [72]. The Pathway-2 trial shows spironolactone's superior efficacy as a fourth-line treatment compared to other antihypertensives. Spironolactone may also benefit obese patients with high sodium intake [72]. ACE inhibitors can cause hypotension, particularly in volume-depleted patients or those on low-sodium diets but may worsen renal function. Other side effects include a persistent dry cough, hyperkalemia, and rare angioedema [73]. Spironolactone, a potassium-sparing diuretic, can lead to hyperkalemia, which poses risks of cardiac arrhythmias [74]. It can also cause gynecomastia, menstrual irregularities, electrolyte imbalances, and potential kidney function deterioration [75, 76]. Severe hyperkalemia occurs in less than 1% of patients after 40 weeks, but potassium levels between 5.5–5.9 mmol/L are more common, especially in those with pre-existing conditions [77]. Careful monitoring of potassium levels and kidney function is essential. Recent advancements in antihypertensive therapy have been limited, with no major new drug targets identified. The focus has shifted to developing combination pills and evaluating new agents like fimasartan (selective for AT1R) and AGSCT101. Fimasartan, an Ang II receptor antagonist, has shown promise in reducing BP and atherosclerotic inflammation, while AGSCT101 is being tested against carvedilol, though detailed information on its efficacy is sparse [78].

Additionally, the introduction of angiotensin receptor neprilysin inhibitors (ARNIs) represents a significant advancement in the treatment landscape for hypertension. ARNIs enhance the levels of natriuretic peptides, which are crucial for promoting natriuresis (the excretion of sodium in urine) and vasodilation. One notable example, LCZ696 (Entresto), demonstrates efficacy in hypertensive patients by utilizing neprilysin to inhibit the degradation of atrial natriuretic peptide (ANP) and brain natriuretic peptide (BNP). This mechanism is particularly beneficial for salt-sensitive patients [79]. Clinical trials have shown that LCZ696 offers significantly superior blood pressure control compared to traditional first-line antihypertensive agents, such as valsartan and olmesartan [80, 81]. While diuretics are effective in lowering blood pressure in individuals consuming high-salt diets, they can also lead to adverse effects, including low potassium levels and elevated uric acid, necessitating careful clinical management [82].

4.2 Heart failure

HTN is a leading global risk factor for cardiovascular diseases (CVDs) and mortality. According to the Global Burden of Disease study, HTN is the top cause of CVD-related deaths, responsible for 10.4 million deaths and 21.8 million disability-adjusted life years. Heart failure, resulting from the heart's inability to meet metabolic demands due to reduced cardiac output, often triggers the RAS as a compensatory mechanism. Chronic RAAS activation can lead to cardiac hypertrophy, myocardial fibrosis, ventricular arrhythmias, and ischemic lesions [83]. Elevated bp significantly increases the risk of ischemic heart disease, with a six-fold higher likelihood of myocardial infarction [84]. HTN worsens these conditions by increasing left ventricular (LV) afterload and peripheral resistance, leading to LV hypertrophy, which may be concentric (wall thickening) or eccentric (chamber enlargement). Prolonged hypertension can progress to diastolic dysfunction and heart failure [84]. LV remodeling in hypertension varies with conditions such as diabetes or high SBP.

4.2.1 Diabetes, RAAS and cardiovascular consequences

Type 2 diabetes significantly disrupts the RAAS, which can be categorized into two main components: the circulating RAAS and the local RAAS. The circulating RAAS regulates systemic blood pressure and fluid balance, while the local RAAS operates within specific tissues, such as the heart and kidneys, and contributes to localized pathophysiological changes [85]. In the classical circulating RAAS, ACE converts Ang I into Ang II—which drive cardiovascular changes [86]. In diabetes, elevated Ang II worsens insulin resistance, leading to increased oxidative stress and inflammation. High blood glucose promotes advanced glycation end-products (AGEs), which further exacerbate oxidative stress and stimulate RAAS components [87, 88]. This cascade results in heightened RAAS activity, promoting hypertension and endothelial dysfunction [89]. Moreover, Diabetes also increases the expression of RAAS components such as ACE and AT1 receptors, intensifying Ang II's harmful effects. Renal renin secretion rises, elevating Ang I and, with increased ACE activity, Ang II levels. Oxidative stress and inflammatory cytokines further activate ACE, increasing Ang II production. Elevated Ang II, through transcription factors NF-kB and AP-1, enhances AT1 receptor expression, thereby intensifying vasoconstriction, inflammation, and fibrosis.

In contrast, local RAAS activity, driven by systemic Ang II and local renin release, contributes significantly to harmful cardiac remodeling, while sympathetic nervous system overactivity promotes further renin release and AT1 receptor expression [88]. Here, the role of the counterregulatory axis, particularly Ang (I–VII) and ACE2, becomes crucial. Ang (I–VII) binds to the Mas receptor, a G protein-couples receptor that mediates various beneficial cardiovascular effects. The Mas receptor involved in vasodilation, anti-inflammatory responses, and the inhibition of cell growth and fibrosis, counteracting the harmful effects of Ang II. Through its activation, Ang (I–VII) promoted cardioprotective mechanism, reducing cardiac fibrosis and hypertrophy and ultimately providing cardiovascular protection [90, 91]. In diabetic cardiomyopathy, excessive Ang II induces cardiac remodeling by stimulating fibroblast activity and collagen deposition, whereas Ang (I–VII) counteracts these effects [89]. In vitro studies have shown that Ang (I–VII) improves cardiac hypertrophy and diastolic dysfunction while reducing oxidative stress [92]. Additionally, mice lacking ACE2 show reduced systolic function [5]. Studies such as the Micro-HOPE trial, highlight that ACE inhibitors can lower cardiovascular risks in diabetic patients, emphasizing the need to target RAAS dysregulation [93]. Despite these findings, the existing literature lacks a critical perspective on the balance between Ang II and Ang (I–VIII), particularly in how local RAAS activity can be leveraged for therapeutic interventions. While ACE inhibitors and Ang II receptor blockers have been established as effective treatments, exploring the therapeutic potential of targeting local RAAS components and enhancing Mas receptor signaling could offer novel strategies for managing cardiovascular complications in diabetes. Overall, the intricate relationship between circulating and local RAAS in diabetes establishes a feedback loop of increased Ang II and AT1 receptor activity, raising cardiovascular risk and contributing to hypertension, heart failure, and related complications.

4.2.2 Atherosclerosis, RAAS and heart failure

Cardiac remodeling, as defined by Cohn et al., involves genetic, molecular, cellular, and interstitial changes that significantly impact the heart's size, shape, and function following cardiac injury [94]. This process includes left ventricular hypertrophy (LVH), which is particularly relevant in atherosclerosis as myocardial infarction (MI) often follows atherosclerotic plaque rupture and subsequent thrombotic events [95]. Atherosclerosis reduces coronary blood flow due to plaque accumulation, leading to MI and is a primary cause of cardiovascular diseases [96–98]. When myocardial cells are damaged by inadequate blood supply, a repair process involving cardiac remodeling and LVH is triggered, driven by hemodynamic stress and the activation of the RAAS [94]. Ang II, a key RAAS mediator, exacerbates myocardial hypertrophy through AT1R, increasing cardiomyocyte size and altering gene expression to favor protein synthesis [99]. Studies show that AT1R antagonists can mitigate Ang II-induced hypertrophy, highlighting the RAAS's role in atherosclerosis and cardiac remodeling [24]. In atherosclerotic plaques, the RAAS is notably active with elevated ACE, Ang II, and AT1R levels [24, 100]. This interplay demonstrates how atherosclerosis-induced RAAS activation leads to significant cardiac alterations, contributing to heart failure. Cardiac fibrosis, marked by excessive extracellular matrix (ECM) protein deposition, exacerbates heart failure and is closely linked with atherosclerosis, as MI from plaque rupture can initiate fibrosis [95, 101]. Ang II interacts with AT1Rs on cardiac fibroblasts, activating fibrogenic pathways such as upregulation of Transforming Growth Factor-β (TGF-β) and myofibroblast activation [102–104]. These processes involve Smad-dependent and Smad-independent pathways, regulated by microRNAs. Additionally, Ang II activates STAT3, enhancing ECM production and promoting fibrosis through collagen synthesis and myofibroblast differentiation [105]. RAAS activation following atherosclerotic plaque rupture not only drives myocardial fibrosis but also impairs cardiac function, underscoring its critical role in cardiovascular disease progression. Elevated BP from atherosclerosis leads to chronic RAAS activation, promoting excessive extracellular matrix (ECM) deposition and myocardial stiffness [106]. This stiffness impairs myocardial relaxation, contributing to diastolic dysfunction and reduced cardiac output. Atherosclerosis-induced hypertension accelerates fibrosis, replacing functional myocardium with non-contractile scar tissue and leading to heart failure. Additionally, fibrosis disrupts normal electrical conduction, increasing susceptibility to arrhythmias, which are common in advanced heart failure.

4.2.3 Mechanisms of RAAS overactivity in heart failure and its clinical management

The overactivation of RAAS is central to the progression of heart failure, with ACE inhibitors (ACE-I), ARBs, and MRAs forming essential components of current HF treatment strategies [8]. Importantly, systemic RAAS and local angiotensin pathways in tissues operate independently, as changes in systemic and tissue-derived angiotensin during HF often do not align. Notably, cardiac Ang II levels are approximately 100 times higher than plasma levels, likely due to intrinsic cardiac Ang I production, which constitutes a significant portion of cardiac Ang II synthesis [107]. In HF, the balance is further disrupted by heightened ACE/ACE2 ratios and intracellular chymase activity, both of which contribute to increased Ang II production via both ACE-dependent and chymase-dependent pathways within the heart [108, 109]. Intracellular sources of Ang (I–XII) and chymase, found in various cell types including mast cells and cardiac fibroblasts, further enhance Ang II generation in HF, potentially exacerbating cardiac dysfunction and remodeling [110, 111]. Conversely, ACE2 exerts cardioprotective effects by counteracting Ang II actions, with its activity regulated by sheddases such as ADAM 17, which are located near ACE2 in the cellular membrane and their activation results in the secretion of a soluble form of tissue ACE2 into the circulation and decreases its activity in the heart [112, 113]. This intricate interplay between circulating and local RAAS components highlights critical therapeutic targets for mitigating HF progression. Future research should aim to further elucidate these mechanisms, explore novel treatment approaches, and address the complex relationships between systemic and local RAAS activities in heart failure.

4.2.4 Advancements in RAAS-targeted therapy for cardiovascular disorders: Clinical evidence and future directions

Clinical trials have shown that RAAS-targeting drugs, including ACE inhibitors (ACEIs) and angiotensin receptor blockers (ARBs), are effective in managing cardiovascular conditions beyond hypertension. ACEIs, such as enalapril and lisinopril, reduce morbidity and mortality in heart failure and post-myocardial infarction patients by decreasing afterload, preload, and systolic wall stress, thereby improving cardiac output without affecting heart rate [114]. Randomized trials consistently demonstrate their significant impact on reducing mortality in heart failure patients with reduced ejection fraction and asymptomatic left ventricular dysfunction, establishing them as the preferred initial therapy [115]. The SOLVD trial highlighted that ACEIs alleviate symptoms, reduce hospitalizations, and lower mortality rates in heart failure patients [116]. However, ACEIs can cause transient renal function decline, dry cough, and hyperkalemia, particularly in patients with kidney issues or diabetes [116–119].

Calcium channel blockers (CCBs), such as amlodipine and verapamil, also significantly affect left ventricular hypertrophy (LVH) beyond their BP-lowering effects. CCBs reduce LVH by inhibiting calcium influx into myocardial cells, while ACEIs and ARBs prevent hypertrophic effects by blocking Ang II formation or its receptor [120]. These medications may lead to complications like peripheral edema and hypotension, necessitating careful monitoring [121]. RAAS activation contributes to vasoconstriction, cardiac and vascular hypertrophy, and fibrosis, leading to cardiovascular and renal complications. While RAAS blockade with ACEIs and ARBs is effective in hypertension, acute myocardial infarction, and heart failure, combining these drugs can increase the risk of hypotension and hyperkalemia, with studies like ONTARGET showing conflicting outcomes [65]. Recent research challenges the notion that LVH is irreversible, indicating that ACEIs, ARBs, and CCBs can improve LVH, with ARBs particularly effective in regression [122, 123].

Advancements in RAAS-targeted therapy include ARNIs, which combine an ARB with a neprilysin inhibitor, such as valsartan and sacubitril. ARNIs increase natriuretic peptide levels, promoting natriuresis, vasodilation, and improved cardiac function. Landmark trials, including PARADIGM-HF and PARAGON-HF, demonstrate that ARNIs significantly reduce cardiovascular mortality and hospitalizations for heart failure by 25–30% compared to traditional ACEIs or ARBs [124, 125].

Research shows that LVH regression is more common in younger patients and correlates with reductions in systolic blood pressure (SBP). However, reversing LVH becomes more challenging with prolonged hypertension due to fibrous remodeling [126–128]. Early detection and effective treatment of hypertension are essential, as LVH may become irreversible over time [128]. RAAS modulators, including ACEIs, ARBs, mineralocorticoid receptor blockers (MRBs), and newer direct renin inhibitors, remain central to managing various cardiovascular disorders. Evidence suggests that dual inhibition of neprilysin and the AT1 receptor using ARNIs can effectively reduce SBP and prevent the development of LV hypertrophy, fibrosis, and both systolic and diastolic dysfunction [129]. While ARNIs are primarily indicated for heart failure patients with reduced ejection fraction (HF-REF), their application in chronic kidney disease (CKD) remains a topic of ongoing debate [130]. Continued research and personalized treatment approaches are vital for optimizing outcomes for patients at risk of cardiac remodeling and dysfunction.

4.3 Renal dysfunction

Chronic kidney disease (CKD) has emerged as a significant global public health concern, with prevalence rates increasing to 8–16% among adults worldwide over the past two decades [131]. CKD is characterized by a persistent decline in glomerular filtration rate (GFR), which measures the volume of fluid filtered from the glomerular capillaries into Bowman's capsule. A GFR below 0.06 L/min for more than 3 months indicates impaired kidney function. This decline is associated with reduced renal blood flow, activating stretch receptors in the arteriolar arteries and dense plaques, which initiates increased renin secretion and triggers the renin-angiotensin-aldosterone system (RAAS) [132]. The RAAS plays a crucial role in maintaining renal blood flow and GFR through the actions of angiotensin II (Ang II) and angiotensin III (Ang III), which induce vasoconstriction and stimulate aldosterone secretion, leading to sodium and water retention. This accumulation of toxins and elevation in hemodynamic load exacerbates CKD progression and fosters cardiovascular complications related to fluid overload and electrolyte imbalance [133].

Elevated BP is both a cause and consequence of CKD. The interplay between hypertension and CKD is complex, involving multiple pathways that contribute to renal damage and disease progression. Epidemiological studies consistently demonstrate a direct relationship between elevated BP and the incidence of CKD across various populations [9]. The kidneys regulate BP through sodium and water balance, renin secretion, and modulation of vascular tone. When BP is chronically elevated, these regulatory mechanisms are disrupted, leading to structural and functional changes in the kidneys.

4.3.1 Mechanisms of hypertension-induced kidney damage

The pathophysiology of hypertension-induced kidney damage involves several interconnected mechanisms. Firstly, systemic hypertension imposes increased pressure on the glomerular capillaries, a condition referred to as glomerular hypertension. In a healthy kidney, the glomerular capillaries are uniquely designed to filter blood under regulated pressure. However, sustained elevation in systemic BP disrupts this delicate balance, leading to increased intraglomerular pressure [134]. This elevated pressure directly stresses the glomerular filtration barrier, composed of endothelial cells, the glomerular basement membrane, and podocytes. Over time, this mechanical strain induces structural changes such as thickening of the glomerular basement membrane and podocyte injury, compromising their function in maintaining glomerular filtration. Secondly, hypertension-induced kidney damage is exacerbated by endothelial dysfunction and impaired autoregulation within the kidney vasculature [135]. Endothelial dysfunction refers to a state where the endothelial cells lining the blood vessels lose their normal function, leading to impaired vasodilation and increased vascular permeability. In the context of hypertension, endothelial dysfunction occurs due to oxidative stress, inflammation, and reduced nitric oxide bioavailability. These factors not only impair vasodilation but also promote vasoconstriction and endothelial cell activation, further contributing to increased vascular resistance and elevated systemic BP [135].

4.3.2 Diabetes, RAAS and kidney disease

Diabetic nephropathy (DN) is a prevalent complication of diabetes mellitus, leading to significant structural and functional disruptions in the kidneys. Research indicates that glucose stimulates growth factors like Ang II and transforming growth factor-beta (TGF-β) in tubular and glomerular cells, likely through oxidative stress [136]. Initial manifestations of diabetic kidney damage include glomerular enlargement and basement membrane abnormalities, which progress to various nonspecific changes such as arteriolar hyalinization, glomerulosclerosis, tubular atrophy, interstitial inflammation, and fibrosis [136]. Chronic hyperglycemia promotes the production of humoral mediators and cytokines in renal cells, accelerating the formation of advanced glycation end-products (AGEs), a key contributor to atherosclerosis in diabetics. This process impairs cell growth and exacerbates glomerular and tubular damage, advancing kidney disease [137].

Ang II, synthesized in the kidneys, plays a crucial role in DN progression. Although the activation of the RAAS is well-documented in diabetes, the specific effects of hyperglycemia on RAAS components remain contentious. Day et al. reported increased intrarenal Ang I and Ang II, alongside elevated levels of AT1R and AT2R in diabetic mice kidneys [136], while Xue et al. observed heightened angiotensinogen (AGT) mRNA but reduced ACE and AT1R mRNA in diabetic rat kidneys [137]. Hyperglycemia activates the RAAS by increasing AGT expression, enhancing renin release, and decreasing ACE2 activity, leading to elevated Ang II levels [138]. Elevated Ang II contributes to glomerular hypertension, oxidative stress, and inflammation, promoting podocyte injury, mesangial expansion, and tubulointerstitial fibrosis. Additionally, hyperglycemia induces epithelial-mesenchymal transition (EMT) in renal epithelial cells, which is crucial for renal fibrosis and DN progression.

These findings highlight the intricate relationship between hyperglycemia, RAAS activation, and EMT in diabetic kidney disease, suggesting potential therapeutic targets [138]. AGEs also modify low-density lipoprotein (LDL), causing cholesterol accumulation in macrophages and foam cell formation, which aggravates endothelial dysfunction and inflammation, thereby accelerating atherogenesis. The interaction between renal function and atherosclerosis in diabetes is reciprocal: diabetes accelerates both atherosclerosis and CKD, while impaired renal function further exacerbates atherosclerosis, establishing CKD as a significant, independent risk factor for atherogenesis [139].

4.3.3 Atherosclerosis, RAAS and kidney disease

End-stage renal disease (ESRD) is a significant concern due to its progression being linked to cardiovascular diseases (CVDs), particularly atherosclerosis, a leading cause of morbidity and mortality in chronic kidney disease (CKD) [140]. Up to 30% of CKD patients have atherosclerotic plaques, with atherosclerotic renal vascular disease (ARVD) being a common cause in Western societies [141, 142]. Additionally, 50% of those with atherosclerosis exhibit renal artery changes, and 6.8% of adults over 65 experience significant renal artery stenosis (≥60%) [143].

Atherosclerosis develops through complex cellular and molecular responses to various insults, with early events resembling those in CKD. Glomerular cells share features with vascular wall cells, suggesting a similarity between atherosclerosis and glomerulosclerosis [144, 145]. Atherogenic lipoproteins, such as oxidized low-density lipoprotein (ox-LDL), induce dysfunction in endothelial and epithelial cells, infiltrate the mesangium and blood vessels, and stimulate growth factor release. This cascade results in glomerular and vascular hypercellularity and extracellular matrix (ECM) proliferation, key pathological features of both conditions [144].

Hypertension affects most CKD patients, with prevalence increasing as glomerular filtration rate declines [146]. Even mild-to-moderate hypertension significantly accelerates CKD progression, and the prehypertensive state correlates with elevated inflammatory markers associated with atherosclerosis [147]. The renin-angiotensin-aldosterone system (RAAS), particularly through angiotensin II (Ang II), plays a crucial role in atherosclerosis. Ang II initiates cellular signaling that exacerbates endothelial dysfunction and oxidative stress via NADPH oxidase, generating reactive oxygen species (ROS) such as superoxide anions (O_2^-) [148]. Increased Nox5 expression further amplifies oxidative and inflammatory responses in vascular cells and macrophages [149].

Activation of the RhoA/ROCK pathway and subsequent MAPK activation lead to nuclear factor kappa B (NF-κB) activation, orchestrating pro-inflammatory cytokine expression and adhesion molecule upregulation, which drive mononuclear leukocyte migration and vascular inflammation [148]. Ang II also enhances LOX-1 receptor expression, increasing oxLDL uptake and foam cell formation, worsening endothelial dysfunction and vascular inflammation [150]. Increased blood pressure causes mechanical stretching in arterial walls, triggering Ang II production, ROS formation, growth factor activation, and ECM proliferation, all vital in vascular remodeling and atherogenesis [151]. Collectively, these mechanisms highlight the critical need to target the RAAS in therapeutic strategies for managing both cardiovascular and renal diseases [106].

4.3.4 Renal function and CKD progression: Insights into RAAS inhibition and innovative therapies

The progression of chronic renal insufficiency is driven by complex mechanisms affecting glomerular filtration rate (GFR) and renal perfusion pressure. Moderate reductions in perfusion pressure and blood flow can decrease GFR, but early adaptations in kidney oxygenation can mitigate severe hypoxia and prevent irreversible damage [152]. Early intervention is beneficial in preserving renal function and delaying fibrosis. A significant advancement in managing chronic kidney disease (CKD) was the identification of the renin-angiotensin-aldosterone system (RAAS) in the early 1990s. Clinical trials have shown that ACE inhibitors and angiotensin II AT1 receptor blockers can slow CKD progression, though they do not completely halt it [153]. In diabetic kidney disease, medications like captopril and losartan have been shown to slow functional decline compared to placebo, but this decline remains faster than age-related loss alone [154]. Current management of renal artery stenosis often favors observation over revascularization for moderate cases with negative scintigraphy results, focusing on monitoring and addressing dyslipidemia and hypertension with ACE inhibitors or ARBs [155]. However, these treatments can lead to elevated serum creatinine and hyperkalemia, necessitating alternatives like calcium channel blockers [156].

Studies have highlighted the potential benefits of angiotensin receptor-neprilysin inhibitors (ARNIs) in managing kidney health alongside heart failure. In the PARADIGM-HF trial, sacubitril/valsartan demonstrated a smaller decline in estimated GFR and reduced composite kidney events compared to traditional therapies [157]. Similarly, PARAGON-HF showed that ARNIs could mitigate adverse kidney outcomes without affecting the progression to end-stage renal disease (ESRD) [158]. However, some studies found no significant differences in kidney function between ARNI and ARB treatments in CKD patients, suggesting that ARNIs may not provide additional benefits over ACE inhibitors or ARBs in this population [159]. Nevertheless, ARNIs are recognized as a promising first-line therapy for heart failure patients, particularly those with reduced ejection fraction (HF-REF) and concurrent CKD, emphasizing the importance of personalized treatment approaches and careful monitoring for side effects.

Future CKD management aims to explore enzymatic processes affecting angiotensin metabolism in the kidneys, with recent studies highlighting potential targets like chymase inhibitors to rebalance angiotensin levels and reduce renal damage [153].

Proteinuria, a key marker of nephropathy, independently predicts CKD progression and cardiovascular risk. Targeting the RAAS has been effective in reducing proteinuria and slowing CKD progression, particularly in diabetic patients and those with mild to moderate CKD [160]. Trials such as RENAAL and IDNT demonstrated significant reductions in proteinuria and renal risk outcomes with losartan and irbesartan, establishing them as first-line therapies for proteinuric CKD [161]. However, as CKD advances, patients face diminished quality of life and increased risks of renal-replacement therapy, cardiovascular events, and mortality [162–164]. Limited evidence suggests that discontinuing RAAS inhibitors may improve estimated GFR in these patients [165]. Ongoing research and clinical trials are crucial for enhancing understanding of CKD pathophysiology and optimizing treatment strategies, with future efforts focused on uncovering additional mechanisms and new therapeutic targets to improve patient outcomes.

5. Future perspective and conclusion(s)

This chapter highlights the critical role of the renin-angiotensin-aldosterone system (RAAS) in maintaining cardiovascular and renal health. By regulating blood pressure, cardiac function, and kidney performance, RAAS is integral to conditions such as hypertension, heart failure, and chronic kidney disease (CKD). Clinical trials have demonstrated that RAAS inhibitors, including ACE inhibitors and angiotensin receptor blockers (ARBs), effectively reduce morbidity and mortality associated with these diseases, marking significant advancements in nephrology [166, 167].

However, excessive RAAS inhibition—especially through combinations of multiple agents—can compromise renal autoregulation and elevate the risk of acute kidney injury, particularly in older CKD patients [168]. Identifying the optimal level of RAAS inhibition is crucial to maximizing antialbuminuric effects without sacrificing renal perfusion. Adding a second RAAS inhibitor for patients unresponsive to the first has often proven ineffective, underscoring the need for novel nephroprotective therapies like SGLT2 inhibitors and endothelin receptor antagonists, which operate through different mechanisms [169].

Research shows that combining SGLT2 inhibitors with RAAS inhibitors—such as ARNIs and ACE inhibitors—can significantly reduce CKD progression and cardiovascular events while also mitigating the hyperkalemia risk associated with RAAS inhibition [130]. Future strategies must focus on effectively combining these therapies for optimal renal and cardiovascular protection, minimizing side effects. While current combinations show promise, they may still pose risks for some patients, highlighting the importance of personalized treatment approaches.

Understanding the mechanisms of kidney damage in CKD is vital for tailored care. Biomarkers indicating tubular and glomerular injury could aid in predicting therapy responses [170]. Given RAAS's widespread presence across the brain, kidneys, heart, and vascular system, further exploration of its roles in health and disease is warranted. For example, the ARB losartan has shown potential in inhibiting glioblastoma growth through Ang II/AGTR1 signaling pathways [171].

Recent evidence underscores the importance of endothelial function in peripheral arterial physiology. Impaired flow and oxidative stress can lead to endothelial dysfunction, increasing cardiovascular risk. Targeting vascular inflammation through RAAS blockers and other antihypertensive therapies has proven effective in improving vascular function. Additionally, extracellular vesicles (EVs) offer promising

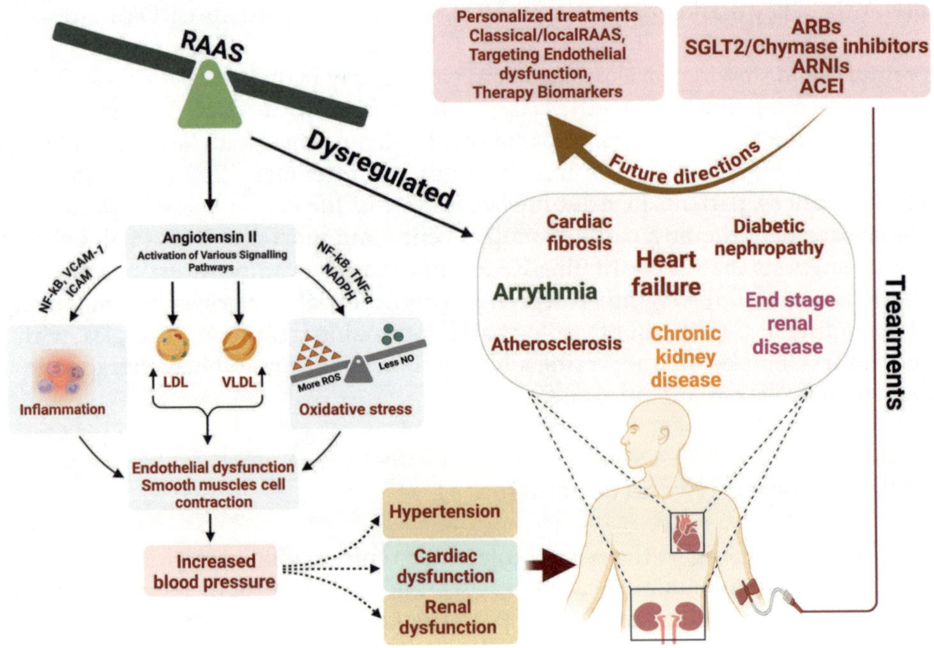

Figure 4.
Impact of dysregulated RAAS on cardiovascular and renal health: current treatments and future directions. This summary figure illustrates the complex interactions within the RAAS and its contributions to hypertension and related complications. It begins with the dysregulation of RAAS, leading to increased production of Ang II. This peptide triggers several inflammatory pathways, including the activation of NF-κB and the release of pro-inflammatory cytokines such as TNF-α, as well as VCAM-1 and ICAM-1. Additionally, Ang II increases levels of low-density lipoprotein (LDL) and very-low-density lipoprotein (VLDL). These events increase oxidative stress, mediated in part by NADPH oxidase, contributing to endothelial dysfunction and resulting in the contraction of smooth muscle cells. This cascade ultimately leads to elevated blood pressure, which is associated with hypertension and subsequent cardiac and renal dysfunction. The figure emphasizes the bidirectional relationship between hypertension, cardiac, and renal dysfunction, highlighting potential treatment strategies including ARBs, chymase inhibitors, ARNIs, and ACEIs. It concludes with a forward-looking perspective on future directions in research aimed at classical/local RAAS system and targeting endothelial dysfunction and addressing the need to develop personalized treatment. RAAS: Renin-Angiotensin-Aldosterone System, NF-κB: Nuclear Factor Kappa B, TNF-α: Tumor Necrosis Factor-alpha, VCAM-1: Vascular Cell Adhesion Molecule 1, ICAM-1: Intercellular Adhesion Molecule 1, SMC, ARBs Angiotensin Receptor Blockers, ARNIs: Angiotensin Receptor Neprilysin Inhibitors, ACE: Angiotensin-Converting Enzyme, NADPH: Nicotinamide Adenine Dinucleotide Phosphate, LDL: Low Density Lipoprotein, VLDL: Very Low-Density Lipoprotein.

opportunities for enhancing endothelial health by delivering bioactive molecules, such as miRNA and drugs that interact with RAAS [135]. Future research should investigate both classical and local RAAS systems, as the latter may provide new therapeutic targets to enhance protective mechanisms or mitigate harmful effects [172]. Furthermore, studying how endothelial dysfunction exacerbates cardiovascular disease in hypertensive patients could reveal potential biomarkers for therapy, guiding more effective treatment strategies (**Figure 4**).

Conflict of interest

The authors declare no conflict of interest.

Author details

Aman Singh[1] and Krishna Singh[2]*

1 Department of Medical Biophysics, Schulich School of Medicine and Dentistry, University of Western Ontario, London, ON, Canada

2 Department of Anatomy and Cell Biology, Schulich School of Medicine and Dentistry, University of Western Ontario, London, ON, Canada

*Address all correspondence to: krishna.singh@uwo.ca

References

[1] Yim HE, Yoo KH. Renin-angiotensin system - considerations for hypertension and kidney. Electrolyte Blood Press. 2008;**6**(1):42-50

[2] Atlas SA. The renin-angiotensin aldosterone system: Pathophysiological role and pharmacologic inhibition. Journal of Managed Care Pharmacy. 2007;**13**(8 Suppl. B):9-20

[3] Ghazi L, Drawz P. Advances in understanding the renin-angiotensin-aldosterone system (RAAS) in blood pressure control and recent pivotal trials of RAAS blockade in heart failure and diabetic nephropathy. F1000Res. 2017;**6**:6

[4] Ichihara A et al. Renal renin-angiotensin system. Contributions to Nephrology. 2004;**143**:117-130

[5] Crackower MA et al. Angiotensin-converting enzyme 2 is an essential regulator of heart function. Nature. 2002;**417**(6891):822-828

[6] Lavoie JL, Sigmund CD. Minireview: Overview of the renin-angiotensin system--an endocrine and paracrine system. Endocrinology. 2003;**144**(6):2179-2183

[7] Kim S, Iwao H. Molecular and cellular mechanisms of angiotensin II-mediated cardiovascular and renal diseases. Pharmacological Reviews. 2000;**52**(1):11-34

[8] Ponikowski P et al. 2016 ESC guidelines for the diagnosis and treatment of acute and chronic heart failure: The task force for the diagnosis and treatment of acute and chronic heart failure of the European Society of Cardiology (ESC) developed with the special contribution of the heart failure association (HFA) of the ESC. European Heart Journal. 2016;**37**(27):2129-2200

[9] Afkarian M et al. Kidney disease and increased mortality risk in type 2 diabetes. Journal of the American Society of Nephrology. 2013;**24**(2):302-308

[10] Nguyen G et al. Pivotal role of the renin/prorenin receptor in angiotensin II production and cellular responses to renin. The Journal of Clinical Investigation. 2002;**109**(11):1417-1427

[11] Touyz RM et al. Vascular smooth muscle contraction in hypertension. Cardiovascular Research. 2018;**114**(4):529-539

[12] Wynne BM, Chiao CW, Webb RC. Vascular smooth muscle cell signaling mechanisms for contraction to angiotensin II and endothelin-1. Journal of the American Society of Hypertension. 2009;**3**(2):84-95

[13] Wang Y et al. Smooth muscle cells contribute the majority of foam cells in ApoE (Apolipoprotein E)-deficient mouse atherosclerosis. Arteriosclerosis, Thrombosis, and Vascular Biology. 2019;**39**(5):876-887

[14] Kim HR et al. Smooth muscle signalling pathways in health and disease. Journal of Cellular and Molecular Medicine. 2008;**12**(6A):2165-2180

[15] Touyz RM. The role of angiotensin II in regulating vascular structural and functional changes in hypertension. Current Hypertension Reports. 2003;**5**(2):155-164

[16] Somlyo AP, Somlyo AV. Ca^{2+} sensitivity of smooth muscle and

nonmuscle myosin II: Modulated by G proteins, kinases, and myosin phosphatase. Physiological Reviews. 2003;**83**(4):1325-1358

[17] Kietadisorn R, Juni RP, Moens AL. Tackling endothelial dysfunction by modulating NOS uncoupling: New insights into its pathogenesis and therapeutic possibilities. American Journal of Physiology. Endocrinology and Metabolism. 2012;**302**(5):E481-E495

[18] Gomez-Garre D et al. Effects and interactions of endothelin-1 and angiotensin II on matrix protein expression and synthesis and mesangial cell growth. Hypertension. 1996;**27**(4):885-892

[19] Vallance P, Collier J, Moncada S. Effects of endothelium-derived nitric oxide on peripheral arteriolar tone in man. Lancet. 1989;**2**(8670):997-1000

[20] Singh A et al. Endothelial-to-mesenchymal transition in cardiovascular pathophysiology. International Journal of Molecular Sciences. 2024;**25**(11):6180

[21] Burckle C, Bader M. Prorenin and its ancient receptor. Hypertension. 2006;**48**(4):549-551

[22] Ramkumar N et al. Renal tubular epithelial cell prorenin receptor regulates blood pressure and sodium transport. American Journal of Physiology. Renal Physiology. 2016;**311**(1):F186-F194

[23] Ramkumar N, Kohan DE. The (pro)renin receptor: An emerging player in hypertension and metabolic syndrome. Kidney International. 2019;**95**(5):1041-1052

[24] Mehta PK, Griendling KK. Angiotensin II cell signaling: Physiological and pathological effects in the cardiovascular system. American Journal of Physiology. Cell Physiology. 2007;**292**(1):C82-C97

[25] Ruiz-Ortega M et al. Role of the renin-angiotensin system in vascular diseases: Expanding the field. Hypertension. 2001;**38**(6):1382-1387

[26] Karnik SS et al. International Union of Basic and Clinical Pharmacology. XCIX. Angiotensin receptors: Interpreters of pathophysiological angiotensinergic stimuli [corrected]. Pharmacological Reviews. 2015;**67**(4):754-819

[27] Touyz RM, Schiffrin EL. Signal transduction mechanisms mediating the physiological and pathophysiological actions of angiotensin II in vascular smooth muscle cells. Pharmacological Reviews. 2000;**52**(4):639-672

[28] Scott JH, Menouar MA, Dunn RJ. Physiology, Aldosterone. Treasure Island (FL): StatPearls; 2024

[29] Stumpe KO, Lowitz HD, Ochwadt B. Fluid reabsorption in Henle's loop and urinary excretion of sodium and water in normal rats and rats with chronic hypertension. The Journal of Clinical Investigation. 1970;**49**(6):1200-1212

[30] Schena M et al. Vasoactive hormones induce nitric oxide synthase mRNA expression and nitric oxide production in human endothelial cells and monocytes. American Journal of Hypertension. 1999;**12**(4 Pt 1):388-397

[31] Touyz RM. Reactive oxygen species and angiotensin II signaling in vascular cells -- implications in cardiovascular disease. Brazilian Journal of Medical and Biological Research. 2004;**37**(8):1263-1273

[32] Kalra D, Sivasubramanian N, Mann DL. Angiotensin II induces

tumor necrosis factor biosynthesis in the adult mammalian heart through a protein kinase C-dependent pathway. Circulation. 2002;**105**(18):2198-2205

[33] Li DY et al. Upregulation of endothelial receptor for oxidized low-density lipoprotein (LOX-1) in cultured human coronary artery endothelial cells by angiotensin II type 1 receptor activation. Circulation Research. 1999;**84**(9):1043-1049

[34] Watanabe T, Barker TA, Berk BC. Angiotensin II and the endothelium: Diverse signals and effects. Hypertension. 2005;**45**(2):163-169

[35] Paffenbarger RS Jr, Thorne MC, Wing AL. Chronic disease in former college students. VIII. Characteristics in youth predisposing to hypertension in later years. American Journal of Epidemiology. 1968;**88**(1):25-32

[36] Boyer JL, Kasch FW. Exercise therapy in hypertensive men. JAMA. 1970;**211**(10):1668-1671

[37] Hackney AC, Lane AR. Exercise and the regulation of endocrine hormones. Progress in Molecular Biology and Translational Science. 2015;**135**:293-311

[38] Nystoriak MA, Bhatnagar A. Cardiovascular effects and benefits of exercise. Frontiers in Cardiovascular Medicine. 2018;**5**:135

[39] Luchner A, Schunkert H. Interactions between the sympathetic nervous system and the cardiac natriuretic peptide system. Cardiovascular Research. 2004;**63**(3):443-449

[40] Tsilosani A, Gao C, Zhang W. Aldosterone-regulated sodium transport and blood pressure. Frontiers in Physiology. 2022;**13**:770375

[41] Chopra S, Baby C, Jacob JJ. Neuro-endocrine regulation of blood pressure. Indian Journal of Endocrinology and Metabolism. 2011;**15**(Suppl. 4):S281-S288

[42] Maggi CA. The mammalian tachykinin receptors. General Pharmacology. 1995;**26**(5):911-944

[43] Landmesser U, Drexler H. Effect of angiotensin II type 1 receptor antagonism on endothelial function: Role of bradykinin and nitric oxide. Journal of Hypertension. Supplement. 2006;**24**(1):S39-S43

[44] Fuchs FD, Whelton PK. High blood pressure and cardiovascular disease. Hypertension. 2020;**75**(2):285-292

[45] Poznyak AV et al. Hypertension as a risk factor for atherosclerosis: Cardiovascular risk assessment. Frontiers in Cardiovascular Medicine. 2022;**9**:959285

[46] Judd E, Calhoun DA. Management of hypertension in CKD: Beyond the guidelines. Advances in Chronic Kidney Disease. 2015;**22**(2):116-122

[47] Gabb G. What is hypertension? Australian Prescriber. 2020;**43**(4):108-109

[48] Dziedziak J et al. Impact of arterial hypertension on the eye: A review of the pathogenesis, diagnostic methods, and treatment of hypertensive retinopathy. Medical Science Monitor. 2022;**28**:e935135

[49] Zhang WW et al. Hypertension and TIA. International Journal of Stroke. 2009;**4**(3):206-214

[50] Zhang Y et al. Associations of blood pressure and cholesterol levels during young adulthood with later cardiovascular events. Journal of

the American College of Cardiology. 2019;**74**(3):330-341

[51] Jia G, Sowers JR. Hypertension in diabetes: An update of basic mechanisms and clinical disease. Hypertension. 2021;**78**(5):1197-1205

[52] Goyal A, Cusick AS, Thielemier B. ACE Inhibitors. Treasure Island (FL): StatPearls; 2024

[53] Singh JN et al. Physiology, Blood Pressure Age Related Changes. Treasure Island (FL): StatPearls; 2024

[54] Iqbal AM, Jamal SF. Essential Hypertension. Treasure Island (FL): StatPearls; 2024

[55] Schmieder RE, Ruilope LM. Blood pressure control in patients with comorbidities. Journal of Clinical Hypertension (Greenwich, Conn.). 2008;**10**(8):624-631

[56] Kalupahana NS, Moustaid-Moussa N. The adipose tissue renin-angiotensin system and metabolic disorders: A review of molecular mechanisms. Critical Reviews in Biochemistry and Molecular Biology. 2012;**47**(4):379-390

[57] Bluher M. Adipose tissue dysfunction contributes to obesity related metabolic diseases. Best Practice & Research. Clinical Endocrinology & Metabolism. 2013;**27**(2):163-177

[58] Dudenbostel T, Calhoun DA. Use of aldosterone antagonists for treatment of uncontrolled resistant hypertension. American Journal of Hypertension. 2017;**30**(2):103-109

[59] Davignon J, Ganz P. Role of endothelial dysfunction in atherosclerosis. Circulation. 2004;**109**(23_suppl_1):III-27-III-32

[60] Ruiz-Ortega M et al. Angiotensin II activates nuclear transcription factor kappaB through AT(1) and AT(2) in vascular smooth muscle cells: Molecular mechanisms. Circulation Research. 2000;**86**(12):1266-1272

[61] Schieffer B et al. Expression of angiotensin II and interleukin 6 in human coronary atherosclerotic plaques: Potential implications for inflammation and plaque instability. Circulation. 2000;**101**(12):1372-1378

[62] Watanabe T, Barker TA, Berk BC. Angiotensin II and the endothelium. Hypertension. 2005;**45**(2):163-169

[63] Chen XL et al. Angiotensin II induces monocyte chemoattractant protein-1 gene expression in rat vascular smooth muscle cells. Circulation Research. 1998;**83**(9):952-959

[64] Kranzhofer R et al. Angiotensin induces inflammatory activation of human vascular smooth muscle cells. Arteriosclerosis, Thrombosis, and Vascular Biology. 1999;**19**(7):1623-1629

[65] Ma TK et al. Renin-angiotensin-aldosterone system blockade for cardiovascular diseases: Current status. British Journal of Pharmacology. 2010;**160**(6):1273-1292

[66] Organization, W.H. Hypertension. Organization, W.H (Geneve, Switzerland). 2023. Available from: https://www.who.int/news-room/fact-sheets/detail/hypertension

[67] Elliott WJ, Ram CV. Calcium channel blockers. Journal of Clinical Hypertension (Greenwich, Conn.). 2011;**13**(9):687-689

[68] Burnier M, Bakris G, Williams B. Redefining diuretics use in hypertension: Why select a thiazide-like

diuretic? Journal of Hypertension. 2019;**37**(8):1574-1586

[69] Sudano I, Roas S, Noll G. Vascular abnormalities in essential hypertension. Current Pharmaceutical Design. 2011;**17**(28):3039-3044

[70] Safar ME, Smulyan H. Atherosclerosis, arterial stiffness and antihypertensive drug therapy. Advances in Cardiology. 2007;**44**:331-351

[71] Nishizaka MK, Zaman MA, Calhoun DA. Efficacy of low-dose spironolactone in subjects with resistant hypertension. American Journal of Hypertension. 2003;**16**(11 Pt 1):925-930

[72] Ghazi L et al. Urinary sodium excretion predicts blood pressure response to spironolactone in patients with resistant hypertension independent of aldosterone status. Journal of Hypertension. 2016;**34**(5):1005-1010

[73] Na, Takuathung M et al. Adverse effects of angiotensin-converting enzyme inhibitors in humans: A systematic review and meta-analysis of 378 randomized controlled trials. International Journal of Environmental Research and Public Health. 2022;**19**(14):2-4

[74] Pongpaew C, Songkhla RN, Kozam RL. Hyperkalemic cardiac arrhythmia secondary to spironolactone. Chest. 1973;**63**(6):1023-1025

[75] Veeregowda SH et al. Spironolactone-induced unilateral gynecomastia. International Journal of Applied & Basic Medical Research. 2018;**8**(1):45-47

[76] Helfer EL, Miller JL, Rose LI. Side-effects of spironolactone therapy in the hirsute woman. The Journal of Clinical Endocrinology and Metabolism. 1988;**66**(1):208-211

[77] Edwards NC et al. The safety and tolerability of spironolactone in patients with mild to moderate chronic kidney disease. British Journal of Clinical Pharmacology. 2012;**73**(3):447-454

[78] Oh M et al. Comparison of fimasartan and amlodipine therapy on carotid atherosclerotic plaque inflammation. Clinical Cardiology. 2019;**42**(2):241-246

[79] Yamamoto K, Rakugi H. Angiotensin receptor-neprilysin inhibitors: Comprehensive review and implications in hypertension treatment. Hypertension Research. 2021;**44**(10):1239-1250

[80] Williams B et al. Effects of Sacubitril/valsartan versus olmesartan on central hemodynamics in the elderly with systolic hypertension: The PARAMETER study. Hypertension. 2017;**69**(3):411-420

[81] Ruilope LM et al. Blood-pressure reduction with LCZ696, a novel dual-acting inhibitor of the angiotensin II receptor and neprilysin: A randomised, double-blind, placebo-controlled, active comparator study. Lancet. 2010;**375**(9722):1255-1266

[82] Garfinkle MA. Salt and essential hypertension: Pathophysiology and implications for treatment. Journal of the American Society of Hypertension. 2017;**11**(6):385-391

[83] Marcy TR, Ripley TL. Aldosterone antagonists in the treatment of heart failure. American Journal of Health-System Pharmacy. 2006;**63**(1):49-58

[84] Levy D et al. The progression from hypertension to congestive heart failure. JAMA. 1996;**275**(20):1557-1562

[85] Kenny HC, Abel ED. Heart failure in type 2 diabetes mellitus. Circulation Research. 2019;**124**(1):121-141

[86] Tipnis SR et al. A human homolog of angiotensin-converting enzyme. Cloning and functional expression as a captopril-insensitive carboxypeptidase. The Journal of Biological Chemistry. 2000;**275**(43):33238-33243

[87] Singh VP et al. Advanced glycation end products and diabetic complications. Korean Journal of Physiology & Pharmacology. 2014;**18**(1):1-14

[88] Chawla T, Sharma D, Singh A. Role of the renin angiotensin system in diabetic nephropathy. World Journal of Diabetes. 2010;**1**(5):141-145

[89] Batista JPT et al. The role of renin-angiotensin system in diabetic cardiomyopathy: A narrative review. Life (Basel). 2023;**13**(7):1598

[90] Donoghue M et al. A novel angiotensin-converting enzyme-related carboxypeptidase (ACE2) converts angiotensin I to angiotensin 1-9. Circulation Research. 2000;**87**(5):E1-E9

[91] Santos RA et al. Angiotensin-(1-7) is an endogenous ligand for the G protein-coupled receptor Mas. Proceedings of the National Academy of Sciences of the United States of America. 2003;**100**(14):8258-8263

[92] Mori J et al. Angiotensin 1-7 ameliorates diabetic cardiomyopathy and diastolic dysfunction in db/db mice by reducing lipotoxicity and inflammation. Circulation. Heart Failure. 2014;**7**(2):327-339

[93] Heart Outcomes Prevention Evaluation Study Investigators. Effects of ramipril on cardiovascular and microvascular outcomes in people with diabetes mellitus: Results of the HOPE study and MICRO-HOPE substudy. Lancet. 2000;**355**(9200):253-259

[94] Cohn JN, Ferrari R, Sharpe N. Cardiac remodeling--concepts and clinical implications: A consensus paper from an international forum on cardiac remodeling. Behalf of an international forum on cardiac remodeling. Journal of the American College of Cardiology. 2000;**35**(3):569-582

[95] Thygesen K et al. Fourth universal definition of myocardial infarction (2018). Circulation. 2018;**138**(20):e618-e651

[96] Severino P et al. Ischemic heart disease pathophysiology paradigms overview: From plaque activation to microvascular dysfunction. International Journal of Molecular Sciences. 2020;**21**(21):8118

[97] Husain K et al. Inflammation, oxidative stress and renin angiotensin system in atherosclerosis. World Journal of Biological Chemistry. 2015;**6**(3):209-217

[98] Nguyen HC, Qadura M, Singh KK. Role of the fatty acid binding proteins in cardiovascular diseases: A systematic review. Journal of Clinical Medicine. 2020;**9**(11):3390

[99] Jugdutt BI. Apoptosis after reperfused myocardial infarction: Role of angiotensin II. Experimental and Clinical Cardiology. 2004;**9**(4):219-228

[100] Dong B et al. Overexpression of ACE2 enhances plaque stability in a rabbit model of atherosclerosis. Arteriosclerosis, Thrombosis, and Vascular Biology. 2008;**28**(7):1270-1276

[101] Bentzon JF et al. Mechanisms of plaque formation and rupture. Circulation Research. 2014;**114**(12):1852-1866

[102] Zeglinski MR et al. TGFbeta1 regulates scleraxis expression in

primary cardiac myofibroblasts by a Smad-independent mechanism. American Journal of Physiology. Heart and Circulatory Physiology. 2016;**310**(2):H239-H249

[103] Wong CKS et al. Connective tissue growth factor expression after angiotensin II exposure is dependent on transforming growth factor-β signaling via the canonical Smad-dependent pathway in hypertensive induced myocardial fibrosis. Journal of the Renin-Angiotensin-Aldosterone System. 2018;**19**(1):1470320318759358

[104] Verjans R et al. MicroRNA-221/222 family counteracts myocardial fibrosis in pressure overload–induced heart failure. Hypertension. 2018;**71**(2):280-288

[105] Han J et al. Angiotensin II causes biphasic STAT3 activation through TLR4 to initiate cardiac remodeling. Hypertension. 2018;**72**(6):1301-1311

[106] Silva GM et al. Role of renin-angiotensin system components in atherosclerosis: Focus on Ang-II, ACE2, and Ang-1-7. Frontiers in Physiology. 2020;**11**:1067

[107] de Lannoy LM et al. Renin-angiotensin system components in the interstitial fluid of the isolated perfused rat heart. Local production of angiotensin I. Hypertension. 1997;**29**(6):1240-1251

[108] Ihara M et al. Increased chymase-dependent angiotensin II formation in human atherosclerotic aorta. Hypertension. 1999;**33**(6):1399-1405

[109] Weber KT, Sun Y. Recruitable ACE and tissue repair in the infarcted heart. Journal of the Renin-Angiotensin-Aldosterone System. 2000;**1**(4):295-303

[110] Ahmad S et al. Primacy of cardiac chymase over angiotensin converting enzyme as an angiotensin-(1-12) metabolizing enzyme. Biochemical and Biophysical Research Communications. 2016;**478**(2):559-564

[111] Patella V et al. Increased cardiac mast cell density and mediator release in patients with dilated cardiomyopathy. Inflammation Research. 1997;**46**(Suppl. 1):S31-S32

[112] Dong B et al. Angiotensin-converting enzyme-2 overexpression improves left ventricular remodeling and function in a rat model of diabetic cardiomyopathy. Journal of the American College of Cardiology. 2012;**59**(8):739-747

[113] Lambert DW et al. Tumor necrosis factor-alpha convertase (ADAM17) mediates regulated ectodomain shedding of the severe-acute respiratory syndrome-coronavirus (SARS-CoV) receptor, angiotensin-converting enzyme-2 (ACE2). The Journal of Biological Chemistry. 2005;**280**(34):30113-30119

[114] Gavras H et al. Angiotensin converting enzyme inhibition in patients with congestive heart failure. Circulation. 1978;**58**(5):770-776

[115] Yancy CW et al. 2017 ACC/AHA/HFSA focused update of the 2013 ACCF/AHA guideline for the management of heart failure: A report of the American College of Cardiology/American Heart Association task force on clinical practice guidelines and the Heart Failure Society of America. Circulation. 2017;**136**(6):e137-e161

[116] Pfeffer MA et al. Effect of captopril on mortality and morbidity in patients with left ventricular dysfunction after myocardial infarction. Results of the survival and ventricular enlargement trial. The SAVE investigators. The

New England Journal of Medicine. 1992;**327**(10):669-677

[117] Murphy BF, Whitworth JA, Kincaid-Smith P. Renal insufficiency with combinations of angiotensin converting enzyme inhibitors and diuretics. British Medical Journal (Clinical Research Ed.). 1984;**288**(6420):844-845

[118] Pinargote P, Guillen D, Guarderas JC. ACE inhibitors: Upper respiratory symptoms. BML Case Reports. 2014:2-6

[119] Perazella MA. Hyperkalemia and trimethoprim-sulfamethoxazole: A new problem emerges 25 years later. Connecticut Medicine. 1997;**61**(8):451-458

[120] Grossman E, Messerli FH. Are calcium antagonists beneficial in diabetic patients with hypertension? The American Journal of Medicine. 2004;**116**(1):44-49

[121] Palmer BF. Managing hyperkalemia caused by inhibitors of the renin-angiotensin-aldosterone system. The New England Journal of Medicine. 2004;**351**(6):585-592

[122] Fagard RH et al. Regression of left ventricular mass by antihypertensive treatment: A meta-analysis of randomized comparative studies. Hypertension. 2009;**54**(5):1084-1091

[123] Chen JS et al. Comparative efficacy of different types of antihypertensive drugs in reversing left ventricular hypertrophy as determined with echocardiography in hypertensive patients: A network meta-analysis of randomized controlled trials. Journal of Clinical Hypertension (Greenwich, Conn.). 2020;**22**(12):2175-2183

[124] Tarun T et al. Updates on new therapies for patients with CKD. Kidney International Reports. 2024;**9**(1):16-28

[125] Anker SD et al. Empagliflozin in heart failure with a preserved ejection fraction. The New England Journal of Medicine. 2021;**385**(16):1451-1461

[126] Chu HW et al. Age-dependent implications of left ventricular hypertrophy regression in patients with hypertension. Hypertension Research. 2024;**47**(5):1144-1156

[127] Lonnebakken MT et al. Left ventricular hypertrophy regression during antihypertensive treatment in an outpatient clinic (the Campania salute network). Journal of the American Heart Association. 2017;**6**(3):1-7

[128] Bang CN, Devereux RB, Okin PM. Regression of electrocardiographic left ventricular hypertrophy or strain is associated with lower incidence of cardiovascular morbidity and mortality in hypertensive patients independent of blood pressure reduction - a LIFE review. Journal of Electrocardiology. 2014;**47**(5):630-635

[129] Stanko P et al. Sacubitril/valsartan alleviates cardiac remodeling and dysfunction in L-NAME-induced hypertension and hypertensive heart disease. Biomedicine. 2024;**12**(4):733

[130] Ksiazek SH et al. Renin–angiotensin–aldosterone system: From history to practice of a secular topic. International Journal of Molecular Sciences. 2024;**25**(7):4035

[131] Taguchi K et al. Uremic toxin-targeting as a therapeutic strategy for preventing cardiorenal syndrome. Circulation Journal. 2019;**84**(1):2-8

[132] Ren L, Lu X, Danser AHJ. Revisiting the brain renin-angiotensin system-focus on novel therapies. Current Hypertension Reports. 2019;**21**(4):28

[133] Ramchandra R et al. Neurohumoral interactions contributing to renal vasoconstriction and decreased renal blood flow in heart failure. American Journal of Physiology. Regulatory, Integrative and Comparative Physiology. 2019;**317**(3):R386-R396

[134] Bidani AK et al. Protective importance of the myogenic response in the renal circulation. Hypertension. 2009;**54**(2):393-398

[135] Gallo G, Volpe M, Savoia C. Endothelial dysfunction in hypertension: Current concepts and clinical implications. Frontiers in Medicine (Lausanne). 2021;**8**:798958

[136] Day RT et al. Acute hyperglycemia rapidly stimulates VEGF mRNA translation in the kidney. Role of angiotensin type 2 receptor (AT2). Cellular Signalling. 2010;**22**(12):1849-1857

[137] Xue H et al. H(2)S inhibits hyperglycemia-induced intrarenal renin-angiotensin system activation via attenuation of reactive oxygen species generation. PLoS One. 2013;**8**(9):e74366

[138] Chen CM, Juan SH, Chou HC. Hyperglycemia activates the renin-angiotensin system and induces epithelial-mesenchymal transition in streptozotocin-induced diabetic kidneys. Journal of the Renin-Angiotensin-Aldosterone System. 2018;**19**(3):1470320318803009

[139] Chade AR, Lerman A, Lerman LO. Kidney in early atherosclerosis. Hypertension. 2005;**45**(6):1042-1049

[140] Collins AJ et al. Chronic kidney disease and cardiovascular disease in the medicare population. Kidney International. Supplement. 2003;**87**:S24-S31

[141] Amann K et al. Special characteristics of atherosclerosis in chronic renal failure. Clinical Nephrology. 2003;**60**(Suppl. 1):S13-S21

[142] Shurrab AE et al. The importance of associated extra-renal vascular disease on the outcome of patients with atherosclerotic renovascular disease. Nephron. Clinical Practice. 2003;**93**(2):C51-C57

[143] Hansen KJ et al. Prevalence of renovascular disease in the elderly: A population-based study. Journal of Vascular Surgery. 2002;**36**(3):443-451

[144] Ross R. Atherosclerosis--an inflammatory disease. The New England Journal of Medicine. 1999;**340**(2):115-126

[145] Kamanna VS, Roh DD, Kirschenbaum MA. Hyperlipidemia and kidney disease: Concepts derived from histopathology and cell biology of the glomerulus. Histology and Histopathology. 1998;**13**(1):169-179

[146] Coresh J et al. Prevalence of high blood pressure and elevated serum creatinine level in the United States: Findings from the third National Health and nutrition examination survey (1988-1994). Archives of Internal Medicine. 2001;**161**(9):1207-1216

[147] Chrysohoou C et al. Association between prehypertension status and inflammatory markers related to atherosclerotic disease: The ATTICA study. American Journal of Hypertension. 2004;**17**(7):568-573

[148] Ziegler T et al. Atherosclerosis and the capillary network; pathophysiology and potential therapeutic strategies. Cells. 2019;**9**(1):3

[149] Touyz RM et al. NOX5: Molecular biology and pathophysiology.

Experimental Physiology. 2019;**104**(5):605-616

[150] Kattoor AJ, Kanuri SH, Mehta JL. Role of Ox-LDL and LOX-1 in Atherogenesis. Current Medicinal Chemistry. 2019;**26**(9):1693-1700

[151] Becker BN et al. Mechanical stretch/relaxation stimulates a cellular renin-angiotensin system in cultured rat mesangial cells. Experimental Nephrology. 1998;**6**(1):57-66

[152] Gloviczki ML et al. Blood oxygen level-dependent magnetic resonance imaging identifies cortical hypoxia in severe renovascular disease. Hypertension. 2011;**58**(6):1066-1072

[153] Laffer CL et al. New insights into the renin-angiotensin system in chronic kidney disease. Circulation Research. 2020;**127**(5):607-609

[154] Lewis EJ et al. The effect of angiotensin-converting-enzyme inhibition on diabetic nephropathy. The collaborative study group. The New England Journal of Medicine. 1993;**329**(20):1456-1462

[155] Fournier T et al. Management of atherosclerotic renal-artery stenosis in 2016. Néphrologie & Thérapeutique. 2017;**13**(1):1-8

[156] Ricco JB et al. How to manage hypertension with atherosclerotic renal artery stenosis? The Journal of Cardiovascular Surgery. 2017;**58**(2):329-338

[157] Damman K et al. Renal effects and associated outcomes during angiotensin-neprilysin inhibition in heart failure. JACC Heart Failure. 2018;**6**(6):489-498

[158] Solomon SD et al. Angiotensin-neprilysin inhibition in heart failure with preserved ejection fraction. The New England Journal of Medicine. 2019;**381**(17):1609-1620

[159] Haynes R et al. Effects of sacubitril/valsartan versus irbesartan in patients with chronic kidney disease. Circulation. 2018;**138**(15):1505-1514

[160] Gansevoort RT et al. Chronic kidney disease and cardiovascular risk: Epidemiology, mechanisms, and prevention. Lancet. 2013;**382**(9889):339-352

[161] Brenner BM et al. Effects of losartan on renal and cardiovascular outcomes in patients with type 2 diabetes and nephropathy. The New England Journal of Medicine. 2001;**345**(12):861-869

[162] Neovius M et al. Mortality in chronic kidney disease and renal replacement therapy: A population-based cohort study. BMJ Open. 2014;**4**(2):e004251

[163] Chronic Kidney Disease Prognosis, C et al. Association of estimated glomerular filtration rate and albuminuria with all-cause and cardiovascular mortality in general population cohorts: A collaborative meta-analysis. Lancet. 2010;**375**(9731):2073-2081

[164] Landray MJ et al. Prediction of ESRD and death among people with CKD: The chronic renal impairment in Birmingham (CRIB) prospective cohort study. American Journal of Kidney Diseases. 2010;**56**(6):1082-1094

[165] Ahmed AK et al. The impact of stopping inhibitors of the renin-angiotensin system in patients with advanced chronic kidney disease. Nephrology, Dialysis, Transplantation. 2010;**25**(12):3977-3982

[166] Bakogiannis C et al. A translational approach to the renin-angiotensin-aldosterone system in heart failure. Annals of Research Hospitals. 2019;**3**:6-11

[167] Ferrari R. RAAS inhibition and mortality in hypertension. Global Cardiology Science and Practice. 2013;**2013**(3):1-10

[168] Riet L et al. Hypertension. Circulation Research. 2015;**116**(6):960-975

[169] de Zeeuw D, Heerspink HJL. Time for clinical decision support systems tailoring individual patient therapy to improve renal and cardiovascular outcomes in diabetes and nephropathy. Nephrology Dialysis Transplantation. 2020;**35**(Suppl. 2):ii38-ii42

[170] Perco P et al. Multimarker panels in diabetic kidney disease: The way to improved clinical trial design and clinical practice? Kidney International Reports. 2019;**4**(2):212-221

[171] Panza S et al. Novel insights into the antagonistic effects of losartan against angiotensin II/AGTR1 signaling in glioblastoma cells. Cancers. 2021;**13**(18):4555

[172] Kanugula AK et al. Renin-angiotensin system: Updated understanding and role in physiological and pathophysiological states. Cureus. 2023;**15**(6):e40725

Chapter 2

The Renin-Angiotensin-Aldosterone System: Mechanisms, Pathophysiological Impacts, and Emerging Therapeutic Strategies

Yan Qing Gong, Hao Liu, Zi Ce Su, Ming Chuan Ba, Xiao Min Li, Li Jun Li and Hong Zhe Zhang

Abstract

The renin-angiotensin-aldosterone system (RAAS) is a pivotal hormonal mechanism integral to cardiovascular and renal homeostasis. This comprehensive review delineates the intricate pathways of RAAS, highlighting its classical and newer axes and their multifaceted roles in physiological and pathological states. We explore the foundational research that has expanded our understanding of RAAS beyond its traditional scope, emphasizing the critical balance between the ACE/Ang II/AT1 axis and the protective ACE2/Ang 1–7/Mas axis. The manuscript delves into RAAS's impact on various organ systems, particularly the cardiovascular and renal, and underscores the system's significance in hypertension, diabetes, and kidney diseases. The review also scrutinizes the therapeutic interventions targeting RAAS, including pharmacological advancements and potential novel approaches. Furthermore, it outlines the challenges and future directions in RAAS-related research, such as personalized medicine, combination therapies, and the development of agonists for the Mas receptor. The evolving landscape of RAAS modulation offers promising avenues for managing complex diseases and emphasizes the need for continued investigation to harness its full therapeutic potential.

Keywords: renin-angiotensin-aldosterone system, angiotensin II, angiotensin-converting enzyme 2, mas receptor, RAAS inhibition, hypertension, cardiovascular protection, diabetic nephropathy, therapeutic targets

1. Introduction

The renin-angiotensin-aldosterone system (RAAS) is a pivotal hormonal system in the human body. Discovered over a century ago, renin was first identified in 1836 when Richard Bright noted the correlation between cardiovascular and renal diseases in his writings, stating, "Cardiac hypertrophy seems to keep pace, to some extent, with the progress of renal disease" [1]. In 1898, Tigerstedt and Bergmann isolated the enzyme renin from the kidneys. Skeggs and colleagues were the first to obtain pure angiotensin. Building on the knowledge provided by these researchers, the study of the role of the renin-angiotensin-aldosterone system in normal and pathological states began, leading to the definition of the classical RAAS pathway in 1961. However, research in this field continues, and studies in the 1990s have proven that the main effector of the RAAS is angiotensin II, which is derived from the progressive proteolysis of angiotensinogen. In addition, angiotensin and aldosterone are also upstream regulatory factors [2]. Over the past few decades, we have seen a considerable expansion of the RAAS. Although it involves multiple organ functions, its primary function seems to have remained largely unchanged. The systemic RAAS cascade begins with angiotensinogen (AGT) produced by the liver, which is converted to angiotensin I (ANG I) by renin secreted by the juxtaglomerular cells of the kidney. Angiotensin-converting enzyme (ACE) secreted by the lungs and kidneys then transforms ANG I into ANG II, while angiotensin-converting enzyme 2 (ACE2) further breaks down ANG II into ANG 1–7 [3].

The primary function of RAAS in altering arterial blood pressure is to regulate peripheral vascular resistance. Angiotensin II exerts its effects through two receptor subtypes, AT1R and AT2R. AT1R mediates the classic actions of ANG II, with AT1 receptors activating neurons in the paraventricular nucleus (PVN), supraoptic nucleus (SON), and medial preoptic area (MnPO) of the hypothalamus, increasing the release of antidiuretic hormone and directly inducing thirst, thereby regulating fluid balance and thirst sensation [4]. Additionally, in terms of excretion, angiotensin, synthesized by Bumpus, Schwarz, and Page in 1957, triggered an in-depth study of the chemistry of angiotensin. Angiotensin II regulates the metabolism of water and sodium by the kidney through direct and indirect effects [5]. Its direct effects include changes in glomerular filtration rate (GFR) and regulation of sodium reabsorption in the renal tubules. By constricting the efferent arterioles, Ang II helps maintain the relative stability of GFR under conditions of hypotension. However, long-term high concentrations of Ang II induce the expression of pro-inflammatory cytokines, such as tumor necrosis factor-α (TNF-α) and interleukin-6 (IL-6), through the activation of signaling pathways like nuclear factor-kappa B (NF-κB). These inflammatory factors can lead to renal tubulointerstitial fibrosis and a decline in renal function, resulting in glomerulosclerosis and a decrease in function [6]. The regulation of sodium reabsorption is achieved by stimulating the sodium-hydrogen exchanger and the sodium-phosphate cotransporter. Ang II stimulates the adrenal cortex to secrete aldosterone, which increases the reabsorption of Na + and the secretion of K+ by promoting the exchange of Na + -K+ in the distal tubules and collecting ducts. Thus, the body maintains a dynamic balance of Na + and K+ concentrations. Vascular resistance is the second factor affecting arterial blood pressure, and angiotensin II itself is one of the most potent vasoconstrictors, activating a series of signaling pathways, including phospholipase C (PLC) and protein kinase C (PKC), leading to an increase in intracellular calcium ion concentration in vascular smooth muscle cells (VSMCs) and activating NADPH oxidase to increase the production of reactive oxygen species (ROS) [7]. ROS promote smooth muscle cell contraction and cause endothelial dysfunction; Ang II can also induce the expression of pro-inflammatory cytokines such as TNF-α, IL-6, monocyte chemoattractant protein 1 (MCP-1), interleukin-1β (IL-1β), and intercellular adhesion molecule 1 (ICAM-1) through the activation of inflammatory signaling pathways, such as the NF-κB pathway [8]. These inflammatory factors can promote the migration of inflammatory cells, exacerbate inflammatory responses, and the proliferation of vascular wall cells; induce the synthesis and secretion of extracellular matrix collagen and fibronectin by vascular smooth muscle cells and fibroblasts, leading to thickening and hardening of the vascular wall, thus causing vasoconstriction.

Angiotensin II (Ang II) exerts various biological effects through its binding to the angiotensin II type 2 receptor (AT2R). Contrary to the proliferative and pro-inflammatory responses mediated by the classic AT1R, the activation of AT2R is generally considered to have a protective effect. The activation of AT2R can cause the relaxation of vascular smooth muscle cells, leading to vasodilation and a reduction in blood pressure. This contrasts with the vasoconstrictive effect mediated by AT1R, inhibiting the production of various pro-inflammatory cytokines, such as TNF-α and IL-6, thereby reducing inflammatory responses; it can inhibit fibrotic reactions, reducing tissue damage and functional loss; it has neuroprotective effects in the nervous system, including reducing neuroinflammation and promoting neurogenesis; in some cases, it has an anti-nociceptive effect, reducing chronic pain by inhibiting neuroinflammation and reducing oxidative stress [8]. The activation of AT2R is generally considered beneficial, and capable of counteracting the harmful effects of Ang II induced by AT1R. These protective effects make AT2R a potential target for the treatment of cardiovascular diseases, kidney diseases, and neurological disorders [9].

The RASS system mainly has two types. One is the ACE/Ang II/AT1 axis, and the other is the ACE2/Ang1–7/Mas axis. They have a significant impact on the cardiovascular system and other physiological systems. This axis consists of angiotensin-converting enzyme 2 (ACE2), angiotensin-(1–7) [Ang-(1–7)], and the Mas receptor (MasR) [9]. Ten years ago, Donoghue et al. [10] discovered ACE's homologous compound ACE2 in the ventricles of patients with heart failure, which has 42% homology in the sequence of the active site with ACE. ACE2 is a zinc-dependent metalloproteinase containing 805 amino acids and is a type 1 transmembrane protein (N-terminus outside the cell, C-terminus inside the cell). It is mainly expressed in vascular endothelial cells and is highly limited to 23 types of tissues, such as the heart, kidney, and intestine [11]. In brain tissue, it can act as a central regulator of cardiovascular function and is mainly distributed in vascular endothelial cells, type I and type II alveolar epithelial cells, pulmonary vascular smooth muscle cells, and bronchial epithelial cells in the lung [12]. ACE2 is also a single carboxypeptidase, removing a single amino acid from the carboxyl terminus of the substrate. Its main substrate is Ang II, and ACE2 can efficiently catalyze the transformation of Ang II into Ang1–7, which is about 400 times more active than hydrolyzing Ang I [13]. When the concentration of Ang I is high, ACE2 can also convert Ang I into Ang1–9, which can be further degraded into Ang1–7 by ACE or other enzymes [14]. Other hydrolysis substrates include Apelin-13, Apelin 36, Neurotensin 1–8, Dynorphin A(1–13), [des-Arg9]-Bradykinin, and [Lys-des-Arg9]-Bradykinin. Ang1–7 is a vasodilatory peptide that, through the Mas receptor, can promote the activation of endothelial nitric oxide synthase (eNOS), increase the concentration of nitric oxide (NO), improve endothelial cell function, reduce pulmonary inflammation, and protect the heart and lungs. This axis is generally considered an antagonistic mechanism of the classical RAS system because of its anti-inflammatory, anti-fibrotic, and anti-proliferative protective effects. ACE2 reduces the level of Ang II by converting Ang II into Ang-(1–7), thus playing a protective role. The Mas receptor is a G protein-coupled receptor that mainly mediates the biological effects of Ang-1-7, causing vasodilation, anti-inflammatory, and antiproliferative effects through the activation of signaling pathways. In recent years, more and more studies have shown that the mutual regulation of the two sub-axes is like the concept of "complementarity of yin and yang, mutual assistance" in Tai Chi (**Figure 1**).

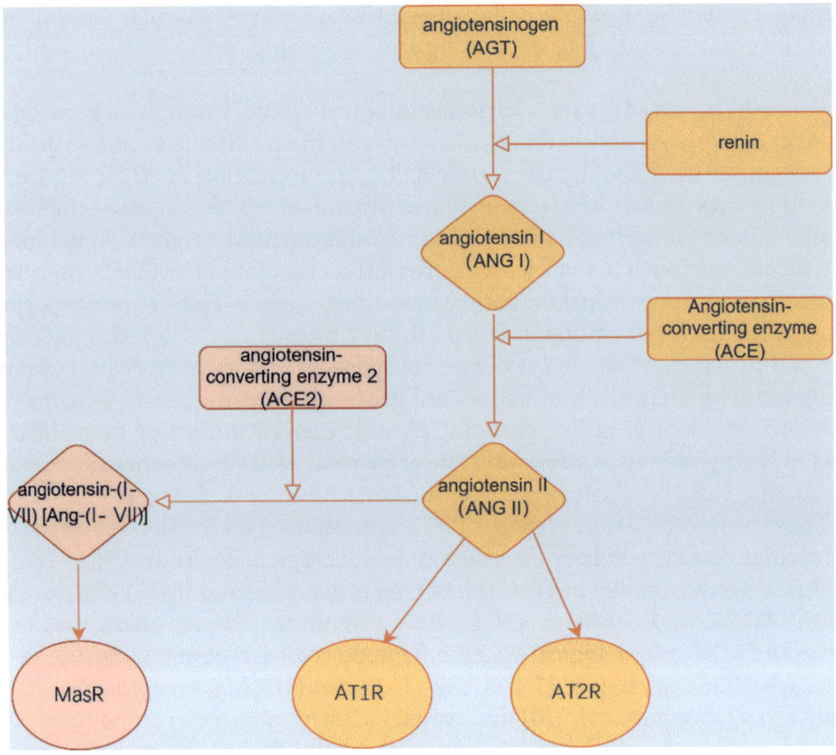

Figure 1.
The Renin-Angiotensin System (RAS) Pathway.

2. The renin-angiotensin-aldosterone system (RAAS) exerts a profound influence on multiple physiological systems, affecting their regulation and balance

This section delves into the multifaceted impacts of RAAS, particularly focusing on its role in the respiratory, circulatory, endocrine, and renal systems.

2.1 Respiratory system

Pulmonary arterial hypertension (PAH) is a critical cause of right heart failure. During the disease process, excessive proliferation and remodeling of pulmonary arterial smooth muscle cells, endothelial dysfunction, imbalance of vasoactive substances, accumulation of perivascular inflammatory cells, and intraluminal thrombosis lead to a gradual increase in pulmonary arterial pressure, inducing right heart failure and functional decline [12, 13, 15]. Damage to pulmonary vascular endothelial cells is considered the initiating link and a necessary condition for pulmonary vascular remodeling [16]. The renin-angiotensin system (RAAS) plays a crucial role in endothelial dysfunction and vascular remodeling. Ang II, through the AT1 receptor, mediates a series of inflammatory reactions, inducing the release of inflammatory cytokines such as IL-6 and TNF-α from vascular endothelial cells and smooth muscle cells. Studies have shown that Ang II also promotes the expression of cell adhesion molecules and chemokines through the activation of the nuclear factor-kappa B (NF-κB) signaling pathway, thereby facilitating the aggregation of inflammatory cells and vascular remodeling [17]. Ang II can also activate the Janus kinase/signal transducer and activator of transcription (JAK/STAT) pathway and transforming growth factor-beta (TGF-β) pathway through oxidative stress and vascular smooth muscle cell proliferation, further promoting myocardial cell hypertrophy and interstitial fibrosis, leading to right ventricular remodeling [18].

In contrast, the ACE2/Ang1–7/Mas axis has a protective role in pulmonary arterial hypertension (PAH). Ang1–7, mediated by the Mas receptor, exerts anti-inflammatory and antiproliferative effects, inhibiting the proliferation and migration of vascular smooth muscle cells, thereby alleviating vascular remodeling. Studies indicate that Ang1–7 can downregulate the expression of inflammatory cytokines (such as IL-6 and TNF-α), suppress the activation of the NF-κB signaling pathway, and reduce inflammatory responses [19]. Additionally, Ang1–7 can alleviate the pathological process of PAH through antioxidant stress and improvement of endothelial function. Other studies have shown that ACE2-transfected human adipose-derived mesenchymal stem cells (ACE2-hAMSCs) significantly enhance migration and angiogenesis capabilities [20]. In a rat model of monocrotaline-induced pulmonary arterial hypertension, transplantation of ACE2-overexpressing hAMSCs resulted in overexpression of ACE2 in lung tissue and downregulation of Ang II expression [9]. ACE2 enhanced the paracrine effects of hAMSCs and promoted blood vessel growth. The expression of factors such as VEGF-a, bFGF, Ang-1, and TGF-β reduced inflammatory factors. At the same time, other studies have shown that Ang1–7 can inhibit myocardial cell hypertrophy and fibrosis through the activation of the Cyclic AMP/Protein Kinase A (cAMP/PKA) signaling pathway [21].

Furthermore, Ang1–7 can alleviate pathological changes by improving myocardial blood flow and oxygen supply. These studies suggest that enhancing the activity of the ACE2/Ang-(1–7)/Mas axis may provide new ideas for the treatment of PAH and right ventricular hypertrophy (RVH). However, further clinical studies are still needed to verify the safety and efficacy of these therapies in humans.

2.2 Circulatory system

2.2.1 Hypertension and heart failure

Hypertension is a common cardiovascular disease caused by the abnormal activation of the RAAS. In hypertension, Ang II activates multiple signaling pathways through the AT1 receptor on myocardial cells, including the extracellular signal-regulated kinases (ERK1/2), Janus kinase/signal transducer and activator of transcription (JAK/STAT), and phosphatidylinositol-3-kinase/protein kinase B (PI3K/AKT) pathways. The activation of these pathways leads to myocardial cell hypertrophy, an increase in cell volume. Ang II can also promote the activation and proliferation of fibroblasts, increasing the deposition of extracellular matrix (ECM), such as collagen, leading to cardiac fibrosis and increased stiffness [22]. These changes can lead to a decrease in cardiac compliance and further promote the progression of myocardial hypertrophy. Ang II regulates the contractility of myocardial cells by affecting intracellular calcium ion concentrations. Abnormal calcium regulation can lead to functional changes in myocardial cells and promote hypertrophy, exacerbating myocardial remodeling [23]. AT1R induces the upregulation of TGF-β through oxidative modification of proteins, lipids, and DNA, destroying cell structures and causing cell death. In particular, NOX2 and NOX4 are highly expressed in myocardial cells and exacerbate myocardial hypertrophy and fibrosis by activating the MAPK and NF-κB signaling pathways, ultimately leading to left ventricular hypertrophy [9].

Studies have shown that ACE inhibitors and Ang II receptor blockers can significantly reduce the levels of inflammatory markers in patients with hypertension, thereby reducing vascular inflammation and remodeling [24]. However, in recent years, a new type of drug, angiotensin receptor-neprilysin inhibitors (ARNIs), has been developed to exert multiple effects by combining angiotensin II receptor blockers (ARBs) and neprilysin inhibitors [25]. The representative drug Sacubitril/Valsartan has shown superior efficacy in the treatment of cardiovascular diseases such as heart failure and left ventricular hypertrophy [26]. In addition to the Valsartan part acting as an ARB, selectively blocking the binding of Angiotensin II to its AT1 receptor, the Sacubitril part also inhibits neprilysin, preventing the degradation of various beneficial peptides (such as natriuretic peptides, vasodilatory peptides, and endorphins) [27]. These peptides help improve heart function through vasodilation, diuresis, reduction of cardiac load, and anti-fibrotic effects. At the same time, these peptides also have antiproliferative and anti-fibrotic effects, preventing myocardial fibrosis and ventricular remodeling. Compared with traditional ARB drugs, the multi-mechanism action on the heart more effectively inhibits myocardial fibrosis, promotes the reversal of myocardial remodeling, and reduces the incidence of cardiac events [28]. Clinical studies, such as the Prospective Comparison of Angiotensin Receptor Neprilysin Inhibitors (ARNI) with Angiotensin-Converting Enzyme Inhibitors (ACEI) to Determine Global Mortality and Morbidity in Heart Failure (PARADIGM-HF) trial, aimed to determine the prognostic performance of B-type natriuretic peptide (BNP) measurements before and during treatment with sacubitril/valsartan. The results of the trial indicated that ARNI significantly outperformed traditional angiotensin II receptor blockers (ARBs) in reducing heart failure hospitalization rates and cardiovascular mortality. In addition to ARNI, other new drugs, such as sodium-glucose cotransporter 2 (SGLT2) inhibitors, have protective effects on the cardiovascular system, especially in hypertension and left ventricular hypertrophy, which has gradually been discovered and studied [29]. The therapeutic mechanism of SGLT2 inhibitors was initially to reduce the reabsorption of glucose in the proximal tubules of the kidney by inhibiting the function of the SGLT2 protein, thereby lowering blood glucose levels. However, in addition to its blood sugar-lowering effect, the protective effects of SGLT2 inhibitors in the cardiovascular system, especially in hypertension and left ventricular hypertrophy, have also been discovered and studied [28]. SGLT2 inhibitors reduce sodium reabsorption in the kidney and increase the excretion of urinary sodium and water retention, leading to a decrease in blood volume, thereby lowering blood pressure. After reducing blood volume and blood pressure, it can reduce the afterload of the left ventricle and alleviate the progression of left ventricular hypertrophy. SGLT2 inhibitors can also increase fatty acid oxidation and ketone body utilization under conditions of limited myocardial oxygen supply, reducing glucose dependence, and placing myocardial cells in a more favorable position in energy metabolism. SGLT2 inhibitors inhibit fibrosis-related signaling pathways (such as the TGF-β pathway) as well as reduce oxidative stress, thereby protecting myocardial structure and function [29]. In addition to these two types of drugs, there are nonsteroidal selective mineralocorticoid receptor antagonists and new anti-fibrotic drugs that can reverse myocardial fibrosis and left ventricular hypertrophy [30].

The protective role of the ACE2/Ang1–7/Mas axis in hypertension has been widely studied. Ang1–7 can promote the release of nitric oxide (NO) by endothelial cells, which is a potent vasodilator. NO binds to soluble guanylate cyclase (sGC), activating the enzyme. Activated sGC catalyzes the conversion of guanosine triphosphate (GTP) to cyclic guanosine monophosphate (cGMP) [24]. cGMP activates protein kinase G (PKG), which further promotes calcium pump activity in the sarcoplasmic reticulum, reducing intracellular calcium concentration and causing smooth muscle relaxation [17, 18, 20]. cGMP can also reduce the sensitivity of smooth muscle cells to calcium through other signaling pathways, further promoting relaxation [26]. In addition, it can increase the production of prostacyclin, further promoting vasodilation and lowering blood pressure. Ang1–7 regulates kidney function through the Mas receptor, inhibiting sodium reabsorption in the renal tubules and promoting the excretion of sodium and water, thereby reducing body blood volume and lowering blood pressure. In the renal tubules, it inhibits the activity of sodium-hydrogen exchanger 3 (NHE3) and sodium-chloride cotransporter (NCC), which are important transport proteins responsible for sodium ion (Na+) reabsorption [22]. When their activity is inhibited, sodium reabsorption in the renal tubules is reduced, and more sodium stays in the tubular lumen to be excreted. It can also reduce the secretion of aldosterone, further inhibiting the reabsorption of sodium by the distal renal tubules and collecting ducts. Ang1–7 inhibits inflammatory reactions by reducing the release of pro-inflammatory cytokines (such as IL-6 and TNF-α), inhibiting myocardial hypertrophy and fibrosis, improving the survival environment of myocardial cells, and protecting myocardial function [22]. Studies have shown that the activation of the ACE2/Ang1–7/Mas axis can significantly reduce the levels of inflammatory markers in patients with hypertension, thereby improving vascular function and structure, reducing left ventricular hypertrophy, and reducing inflammatory reactions and ventricular remodeling.

2.2.2 Coronary atherosclerotic heart disease

In the study of coronary atherosclerosis, the classical RAAS ACE/Ang II/AT1R axis plays a crucial role. This axis promotes the occurrence and development of atherosclerosis through various mechanisms, including oxidative stress, inflammatory reactions, smooth muscle cell proliferation, and extracellular matrix remodeling [31].

Firstly, Ang II is the core effector molecule of the ACE/Ang II/AT1R axis, which activates multiple downstream signaling pathways by binding to its receptor, the angiotensin II type 1 receptor (AT1R). The most critical of these is the oxidative stress response mediated by NADPH oxidase. After binding with AT1R, Ang II activates NADPH oxidase through G protein signal transduction, increasing the production of reactive oxygen species (ROS). ROS further causes endothelial cell dysfunction, increases the permeability of endothelial cells, promotes the oxidation of low-density lipoprotein (LDL), and thus accelerates the formation of atherosclerotic plaques [32]. Secondly, Ang II significantly enhances inflammatory reactions through the NF-κB signaling pathway activated by AT1R. NF-κB is a key transcription factor that plays a central role in inflammation and immune responses. Ang II stimulates the activation of NF-κB, leading to an increase in the expression of inflammatory factors such as IL-6, TNF-α, and MCP-1 [33]. These inflammatory factors further promote the recruitment and adhesion of monocytes, promoting the formation of foam cells and accelerating plaque instability. In addition, Ang II can promote the proliferation and migration of vascular smooth muscle cells (VSMCs) through AT1R. The specific mechanism includes activating the ERK1/2 and p38 MAPK signaling pathways, as well as inducing the expression of early response genes such as Egr-1 and Fos, ultimately leading to the phenotypic transformation of VSMCs from the contractile type to the secretory type. Secretory VSMCs secrete cytokines and growth factors (such as

TGF-β) that can further stimulate the synthesis and deposition of the extracellular matrix, leading to thickening and hardening of the arterial wall. In addition, the ACE/Ang II/AT1R axis also stimulates the secretion of matrix metalloproteinases (MMPs) by endothelial cells and macrophages, causing matrix degradation and vascular remodeling. This process increases the vulnerability of atherosclerotic plaques, making them prone to rupture and thrombosis, thereby inducing acute coronary syndrome [34].

It is worth noting that in addition to the classic AT1R-mediated effects, there is a complex interaction between the ACE2/Ang-(1–7)/Mas axis. The ACE2/Ang-(1–7)/Mas axis plays a role in coronary atherosclerosis through several main mechanisms: 1. Anti-inflammatory effect: Studies have shown that Ang-(1–7) can inhibit the activation of the NF-κB pathway through the Mas receptor, reducing the expression of pro-inflammatory factors such as TNF-α and IL-6, thereby reducing inflammatory reactions. In addition, Ang-(1–7) can also reduce the infiltration of inflammatory cells in the plaque by inhibiting the activation and recruitment of macrophages to the plaque site, thereby lowering the inflammatory state of the plaque. 2. Antioxidant stress: Oxidative stress is an important factor in the occurrence and development of coronary atherosclerosis. Ang-(1–7) can promote the expression of antioxidant enzymes, such as superoxide dismutase (SOD) and catalase, through the Mas receptor-mediated pathway, thereby clearing free radicals and reducing the damage of oxidative stress to vascular endothelial cells and vascular smooth muscle cells. 3. Antiproliferation and anti-fibrotic effects: Ang-(1–7) can inhibit the proliferation and migration of vascular smooth muscle cells through the Mas receptor-mediated signaling pathway, thereby reducing vascular remodeling and plaque formation. In addition, Ang-(1–7) can also reduce the generation and fibrosis of the extracellular matrix by inhibiting the transforming growth factor-beta (TGF-β) and its downstream signaling pathways, thus playing a potential role in the prevention and treatment of coronary atherosclerosis. 4. Vasodilation and improvement of endothelial function: Ang-(1–7) can promote the release of nitric oxide (NO) through the Mas receptor, leading to the relaxation of vascular smooth muscle and improving blood flow dynamics, reducing vascular resistance. In addition, Ang-(1–7) can also improve endothelial cell function, promoting vascular repair and regeneration, thus playing a protective role in coronary atherosclerosis [35].

Although the role of the ACE2/Ang-(1–7)/Mas axis in coronary atherosclerosis has been widely studied, it still faces challenges in clinical application. Currently, several treatment strategies are being explored, including: 1. Ang-(1–7) analogs: The development of stable analogs or receptor agonists of Ang-(1–7) to enhance the protective effect of the ACE2/Ang-(1–7)/Mas axis and delay or reverse the progression of coronary atherosclerosis. These analogs can be delivered through subcutaneous injection, oral administration, or other methods, and research results show that these analogs have good efficacy in animal models. 2. ACE2 enhancers: Increasing the expression or activity of ACE2 through gene therapy or drug intervention to enhance the generation of Ang-(1–7) and play an anti-atherosclerotic role. Recent studies have shown that the exogenous delivery of the ACE2 gene can significantly reduce plaque area and inflammatory reactions in animal models of atherosclerosis. 3. Mas receptor agonists: The development of selective agonists for the Mas receptor to directly activate the downstream signaling pathway of Ang-(1–7), thereby playing an anti-inflammatory, anti-fibrotic, and vascular function improvement role. Several Mas receptor agonists are currently in preclinical research and show potential therapeutic effects. 4. Combined therapy: Considering the opposing roles of the ACE/Ang II/AT1R axis and the ACE2/

Ang-(1–7)/Mas axis in regulating vascular function, some studies have proposed the use of ACE inhibitors or Ang II receptor blockers (ARBs) in combination with ACE2/Ang-(1–7)/Mas axis-related drugs to further enhance the anti-atherosclerotic effect. This combined therapy strategy has shown a certain synergistic effect in clinical research.

In summary, the ACE2/Ang-(1–7)/Mas axis, as a potential therapeutic target for coronary atherosclerosis, has a broad application prospect. However, research on its specific molecular mechanisms and treatment plans still needs further in-depth, especially in large-scale clinical trials.

2.3 Endocrine system

Endocrine system diseases, such as diabetes, Cushing's syndrome, pheochromocytoma, and primary aldosteronism, play a crucial role in the renin-angiotensin system (RAS), especially the molecular mechanisms of the ACE/Ang II/AT1R axis and the ACE2/Ang-(1–7)/Mas axis and their impact on disease progression. With in-depth research on these diseases, people are increasingly recognizing that these two axes represent the pathogenic and protective pathways of the RAS, and their mechanisms of action and potential treatment strategies in various endocrine disorders have become hot topics of current research.

2.3.1 Diabetes

Diabetes is a chronic metabolic disease characterized by hyperglycemia. The ACE/Ang II/AT1R axis plays a key role in the pathogenesis of diabetes. Studies have shown that Ang II interacts with the insulin signaling pathway through AT1R, and leading to the exacerbation of insulin resistance and the apoptosis of pancreatic β-cells. Specifically, Ang II inhibits the IRS-1/PI3K/Akt signaling pathway, disrupting insulin-mediated glucose transport, leading to increased blood glucose levels. In addition, Ang II can also promote the functional decline of β-cells by promoting oxidative stress and inflammatory reactions within β-cells, thereby exacerbating the condition of diabetes. In diabetic nephropathy (DKD), the overactivation of the ACE/Ang II/AT1R axis is the main cause of glomerulosclerosis and interstitial fibrosis of the kidney. Ang II stimulates the proliferation of mesangial cells and the synthesis of extracellular matrix, leading to the occurrence of glomerulosclerosis. In addition, Ang II also promotes the expression of transforming growth factor-beta (TGF-β), promoting the process of interstitial fibrosis. These pathological changes ultimately lead to a decrease in glomerular filtration function, and severe cases can develop into end-stage renal disease (ESRD) [36]. In diabetes, the protective role of the ACE2/Ang-(1–7)/Mas axis is particularly important. Studies have shown that Ang-(1–7) can improve insulin signal transduction through the Mas receptor-mediated effect, reducing insulin resistance. In addition, Ang-(1–7) promotes the generation of nitric oxide (NO), improves endothelial function, and reduces oxidative stress and inflammatory reactions, thereby reducing vascular damage and complications related to diabetes. In diabetic nephropathy, the activity of the ACE2/Ang-(1–7)/Mas axis counteracts the glomerulosclerosis and interstitial fibrosis caused by the ACE/Ang II/AT1R axis. The specific mechanism includes inhibiting the expression of TGF-β, reducing the deposition of extracellular matrix, and maintaining the integrity of kidney structure by inhibiting the proliferation of mesangial cells [37]. Increasing the expression of ACE2 or directly applying Ang-(1–7) analogs is considered a potential strategy for treating diabetic nephropathy. In drug treatment, ACE inhibitors and AT1R antagonists can significantly improve the metabolic state and kidney function of patients by improving insulin sensitivity and slowing the progression of diabetic nephropathy. Especially in patients with diabetic nephropathy, these drugs have become part of the standard treatment to delay the decline of kidney function and reduce proteinuria. In addition to traditional drugs, Dapagliflozin is a selective SGLT2 inhibitor that reduces the reabsorption of glucose by the kidney, thereby lowering blood glucose levels. In addition to its blood-lowering effect, Dapagliflozin also shows a protective effect on the cardiovascular system, especially in diabetic patients. The cardiovascular protective effect of Dapagliflozin is partly related to its regulation of the RAS [35]. Studies have shown that Dapagliflozin can balance the ACE/Ang II/AT1R axis and the ACE2/Ang-(1–7)/Mas axis by reducing the generation of Ang II or enhancing the expression of ACE2, thereby reducing inflammatory reactions, oxidative stress, and fibrosis. These effects are important for preventing cardiovascular complications in diabetic patients, especially heart failure and kidney damage [38]. In clinical practice, Dapagliflozin has been proven to significantly reduce the incidence of cardiovascular events in diabetic patients and delay the progression of diabetic nephropathy. Due to its multiple mechanisms of action, Dapagliflozin is considered a very promising drug for the treatment of diabetes and its complications. In addition to ACE inhibitors, AT1R antagonists, and SGLT2 inhibitors, other drugs targeting the RAS are also showing potential in the treatment of endocrine diseases. For example, direct renin inhibitors (such as Aliskiren) inhibit the activity of renin, reducing the generation of Ang I and Ang II, thereby inhibiting the activity of the RAS. Although the clinical application of these drugs is still being explored, their potential therapeutic value should not be overlooked.

2.3.2 Cushing's syndrome

Cushing's syndrome is an endocrine disease caused by excessive secretion of glucocorticoids. The role of the ACE/Ang II/AT1R axis in Cushing's syndrome is increasingly being paid attention to. Glucocorticoids enhance the activity of the RAAS, especially the activity of the ACE/Ang II/AT1R axis, by upregulating the expression of ACE, increasing the generation of Ang II, and causing a series of adverse reactions through AT1R, including hypertension, insulin resistance, lipid metabolism disorders, and cardiovascular complications. Excessive secretion of glucocorticoids can enhance the activity of the RAAS, especially the activity of the ACE/Ang II/AT1R axis. Ang II causes hypertension in patients with Cushing's syndrome mainly through the vasoconstriction and sodium retention effects mediated by AT1R. In addition, Ang II can also accelerate the progression of atherosclerosis and the increase of cardiovascular events through the oxidative stress pathway. At the metabolic level, Ang II can promote the ectopic deposition of fat by disrupting the function of adipose tissue, thereby exacerbating insulin resistance and glucose metabolism disorders [39]. There is limited research on the ACE2/Ang-(1–7)/Mas axis in Cushing's syndrome, but existing evidence suggests that this axis may play a role in alleviating metabolic disorders and cardiovascular complications caused by excessive glucocorticoids [40]. Ang-(1–7) may counteract the pathogenic effects of the ACE/Ang II/AT1R axis in Cushing's syndrome through its anti-inflammatory and antioxidant effects. In Cushing's syndrome, the expression of ACE is upregulated by glucocorticoids, leading to increased activity of the ACE/Ang II/AT1R axis. Therefore, regulating the activity of the ACE2/Ang-(1–7)/Mas axis to restore the balance of the RAAS may be a promising direction for treatment [41]. Future research needs to further explore the specific mechanisms of this axis in Cushing's syndrome and its therapeutic potential.

2.3.3 Pheochromocytoma and primary aldosteronism

Pheochromocytoma and primary aldosteronism are two common causes of endocrine hypertension. The ACE/Ang II/AT1R axis shows significant activation in these diseases, leading to a marked increase in blood pressure. In pheochromocytoma, due to the secretion of a large amount of catecholamines by tumor cells, the overactivation of the sympathetic nervous system leads to an enhancement of RAAS activity, especially the activity of the ACE/Ang II/AT1R axis. Ang II further exacerbates vasoconstriction and blood pressure increase through the effects of AT1R. In addition, Ang II can also promote the secretion of aldosterone, leading to sodium retention and excessive body fluid, aggravating the degree of hypertension.

Primary aldosteronism is a disease caused by the overproduction of aldosterone by the adrenal cortex. Its main features are refractory hypertension and hypokalemia. Aldosterone leads to an increase in blood volume and elevated blood pressure by increasing sodium reabsorption by the kidney. At the same time, aldosterone can also enhance the activity of the ACE/Ang II/AT1R axis by upregulating the expression of ACE. Ang II, through the vasoconstrictive effects mediated by AT1R as well as by promoting fibrosis and oxidative stress, further exacerbates cardiovascular complications, such as left ventricular hypertrophy and arteriosclerosis. In pheochromocytoma and primary aldosteronism, the role of the ACE2/Ang-(1–7)/Mas axis is also of interest. Studies have shown that Ang-(1–7) can lower blood pressure and reduce cardiovascular complications associated with hypertension through the Mas receptor [42]. In pheochromocytoma, Ang-(1–7) reduces hypertension and cardiovascular complications caused by excessive secretion of catecholamines by inhibiting the pathogenic effects of the ACE/Ang II/AT1R axis. In addition, Ang-(1–7) can also reduce cardiac remodeling and heart failure commonly seen in patients with pheochromocytoma through its anti-fibrotic effects. Studies have found that enhancing the expression of ACE2 or directly applying Ang-(1–7) analogs can significantly improve blood pressure control and cardiovascular prognosis in patients with primary aldosteronism [43]. ACE inhibitors and AT1R antagonists are widely used to control hypertension. By inhibiting the effects of Ang II, these drugs not only effectively lower blood pressure but also reduce the incidence of cardiovascular complications. Especially for patients who cannot undergo surgery, these drugs provide an important noninvasive treatment option. Surgical removal is the preferred method for treating pheochromocytoma, which can usually cure hypertension and other related symptoms completely. Before surgery, patients usually need to control blood pressure with medication to prevent perioperative crises caused by excessive release of catecholamines. Preoperative preparation usually includes the use of alpha-blockers (such as phenoxybenzamine) and beta-blockers (such as propranolol) to stabilize blood pressure and heart rate. In addition, emotional excitement and other factors that may induce the release of catecholamines should be avoided before surgery. After the tumor is removed, most patients' hypertension can be significantly improved or even completely resolved. However, blood pressure and catecholamine levels still need to be monitored after surgery to prevent tumor recurrence or residue [44]. In addition, long-term follow-up after surgery is also crucial for assessing cardiovascular health and preventing complications [45]. Primary aldosteronism is a disease caused by the overproduction of aldosterone by the adrenal cortex, and its main features are refractory hypertension and hypokalemia. Surgical treatment is usually aimed at adrenal cortical adenomas or hyperplasia, and it can restore normal aldosterone levels by removing the affected tissue [36]. For patients with unilateral adrenal adenomas, laparoscopic adrenalectomy is the preferred method. This minimally invasive surgery has a small trauma and fast recovery, and can significantly improve patients' blood pressure and potassium metabolism [46]. Before surgery, patients usually need to control blood pressure and electrolyte balance with medication to reduce complications during and after surgery [47]. For patients with bilateral adrenal hyperplasia, the choice of surgical treatment is more complex and may require individualized treatment based on the patient's specific situation. Long-term follow-up is still needed after surgery to monitor blood pressure and aldosterone levels and adjust drug treatment plans as needed.

2.4 Renal system

Diseases of the renal system are a common group of chronic diseases, among which glomerular diseases, diabetic nephropathy (DN), hypertensive nephropathy (HN), and others are the main types of diseases. The pathogenesis of these diseases is complex and closely related to multiple molecular signaling pathways. The renin-angiotensin system is an important system for regulating renal hemodynamics, salt and water balance, and blood pressure, and its dysregulation plays a key role in the pathological process of kidney diseases.

2.4.1 Diabetic nephropathy

Clinically, acute kidney injury (AKI) is considered a catastrophic disease with high incidence and mortality rates. One of the main risk factors for AKI is diabetes mellitus (DM). Compared with non-diabetic patients, diabetic patients are still at a higher risk of developing AKI [48]. The poor renal outcomes of DM and AKI are mainly attributed to apoptosis, inflammation mediated by NF-κB, and oxidative stress promoted by the renin-angiotensin system (RAS) through mitogen-activated protein kinase (MAPK) [49]. Therefore, inhibiting the RAS with angiotensin II receptor blockers (ARBs) or angiotensin-converting enzyme inhibitors (ACEi) is considered to prevent AKI. Surprisingly, when ARBs and ACEi are used to treat AKI patients, they increase the severity of AKI. This highlights the need for new treatment methods for AKI [35]. The ACE/Ang II/AT1 axis has been deeply explored in the pathophysiology and drug treatment of renal complications, including AKI. However, to date, the role of the ACE2/Ang-(1–7)/Mas axis in the pathogenesis of AKI-DM comorbidity has been little studied. The ACE2/Ang-(1–7)/Mas axis establishes compensatory mechanisms by sensing increased cellular stress and pathological signals, which are beneficial to the renal system. Mice with distal renal injury induced by tourniquet show a disorder of ACE and ACE2 activity, which can lead to kidney damage. Interestingly, restoring the ACE/ACE2 balance by upregulating ACE2 can prevent renal injury. Studies have shown that lipopolysaccharide-induced endotoxemia significantly reduces ACE2 mRNA levels: subsequently, the levels of Ang II and inducible nitric oxide synthase in the kidney are increased, while restoring ACE2 levels can maintain endothelial pore size, glomerular filtration rate, and proximal renal tubular function, ultimately protecting the kidney from AKI. Ruiz-Ortega and others have demonstrated that AT2R is overexpressed in Balb/c renal tubular cells under treatment with folic acid-induced AKI and have put forward the potential role of AT2R in protecting kidney damage [38]. Subsequently, overexpression of AT2R and activation of ACE2 activity significantly improved renal function in these models of mice. Recently, Nisha Sharma and others have shown that inhibiting the ACE2/Ang-(1–7)/Mas axis can induce ischemic AKI in non-diabetic (ND) and streptozotocin-induced diabetic (DM) rats and found that the severity of ischemic AKI is widespread in DM rats, which may be due to the presence of hyperglycemia damage [50]. A new combined therapy targeting the RAAS protective axis with AT2R agonists and ACE2 activators can significantly alleviate systemic and renal RAS changes and prevent renal tubular injury related to IRI in ND and DM rats [51]. Therefore, targeting the ACE2/Ang-(1–7)/Mas axis may be a new therapeutic option for AKI.

2.4.2 Hypertensive nephropathy

Hypertension affects about 30% of the general population. Hypertensive nephropathy is considered one of the complications of long-term and poorly controlled hypertension. Hypertensive nephropathy is the second leading cause of end-stage renal disease (ESRD) after diabetes. Most patients with hypertension will develop mild to moderate hypertensive nephrosclerosis [52]. However, when blood pressure (BP) values are not controlled for a long time or when there is a pre-existing kidney disease, the proportion of patients developing ESRD will increase sharply [53]. For a long time, attention has been paid to renal fibrosis and hyaline degeneration caused by the injury to the glomerular tuft, as well as the activity of the RAS system. However, recently, molecular mechanisms and other histological aspects have been included in the pathophysiology of hypertensive nephropathy, including renal tubular cell injury leading to epithelial-mesenchymal transition (EMT) and renal interstitial fibrosis. Angiotensin II promotes renal oxidative stress and mediates epithelial-mesenchymal transition through the AT1-ERK/mitogen-activated protein kinase (MAP) kinase, TGF-β/Smad2/3, and NF-κB pathways. One of the protective mechanisms of cells against oxidative stress is the production of highly conserved proteins called heat shock proteins (Hsps). Hsps are intracellular proteins that respond to cellular stress and act as chaperon proteins for other "client" peptides, binding to these peptides to prevent their irreversible aggregation and promoting their correct folding, physiological assembly, and intracellular transport. In addition to traditional ACE inhibitors and Ang II receptor blockers (ARBs), treatment strategies based on the ACE2/Ang-(1–7)/Mas axis mainly focus on the development of ACE2 and Mas receptor agonists. ACE2 agonists can inhibit the pathogenic effects of Ang II by increasing the generation of Ang-(1–7) [54]. Currently, ACE2 agonists have shown good renal protective effects in animal models, but their clinical application still needs further verification. Mas receptor agonists play an anti-inflammatory, anti-fibrotic, and antioxidant stress role by directly activating the Mas receptor. The therapeutic potential of these drugs in kidney diseases is also being widely studied. The ACE/Ang II/AT1 axis and the ACE2/Ang-(1–7)/Mas axis play a pathogenic and protective role in hypertensive nephropathy, respectively. With an in-depth understanding of these two signaling axes, more effective treatment strategies can be developed. At present, ACE inhibitors and ARBs have been widely used in clinical practice, and ACE2 and Mas receptor agonists represent a new direction for the treatment of kidney diseases in the future. With in-depth research, these emerging therapies are expected to provide better treatment options for patients with kidney system diseases [55].

2.4.3 Invasive treatment of ACE/Ang II/AT1 axis and ACE2/Ang-(1: 7)/mas axis

The ACE/Ang II/AT1 axis and the ACE2/Ang-(1–7)/Mas axis play a key role in the invasive treatment of the renal system. These axes not only affect the pathological process of the disease but also guide the implementation of certain invasive treatments and their postoperative management.

Renal artery stenosis (RAS) is one of the main causes of renal hypertension and renal insufficiency. The activation of the ACE/Ang II/AT1 axis in RAS leads to a reduction in renal blood flow, which in turn triggers systemic hypertension and renal damage. In this case, renal artery interventional treatment (such as percutaneous renal artery angioplasty or stent implantation) is a commonly used invasive treatment method. This treatment reduces Ang II levels by improving renal artery blood flow, and reducing the pathogenic effects of AT1 receptor-mediated vasoconstriction, inflammation, and fibrosis [56]. Before and after surgery, ACE inhibitors or Ang II receptor blockers (ARBs) are often used in the clinic to further control the activity of the ACE/Ang II/AT1 axis, preventing postoperative hypertension rebound and renal function deterioration. For patients who fail to effectively control blood pressure after surgery, ACE2 agonists and Mas receptor agonists may become potential adjuvant treatment options, further counteracting the harmful effects of Ang II by enhancing the activity of the ACE2/Ang-(1–7)/Mas axis [57].

In patients with end-stage renal disease (ESRD), renal transplantation is the most effective invasive treatment method. However, the transplanted kidney often suffers from acute injury and rejection reactions during reperfusion, and the overactivation of the ACE/Ang II/AT1 axis often exacerbates the damage to the transplanted kidney [58]. Ang II can lead to acute injury and long-term fibrosis of the transplanted kidney by promoting vasoconstriction and inflammation. To reduce these adverse reactions, ACE inhibitors or ARBs are usually required after transplantation to inhibit the activity of the ACE/Ang II/AT1 axis, thereby protecting the function of the transplanted kidney. In addition, the ACE2/Ang-(1–7)/Mas axis also has potential effects in protecting the transplanted kidney after transplantation. ACE2 may help reduce reperfusion injury and inflammatory reactions by reducing the generation of Ang II and increasing the generation of Ang-(1–7). Mas receptor agonists, as a new treatment strategy, may improve the long-term prognosis of the transplanted kidney by activating protective pathways [59]. Hemodialysis treatment, is an important treatment for end-stage renal disease, although not a direct invasive treatment for the kidney, the balance of the ACE/Ang II/AT1 axis and the ACE2/Ang-(1–7)/Mas axis is still crucial during the maintenance of hemodialysis [60]. Hemodialysis patients often have hypertension and cardiovascular diseases, which are closely related to the abnormal activity of the ACE/Ang II/AT1 axis. The use of ACE inhibitors or ARBs can effectively control blood pressure in hemodialysis patients and reduce the incidence of cardiovascular complications.

In summary, the regulation of the ACE/Ang II/AT1 axis and the ACE2/Ang-(1–7)/Mas axis in the invasive treatment of the renal system is of great significance. These axes not only affect the pathological process of the disease but also play a key role in postoperative management and long-term prognosis. In the future, more precise treatment strategies targeting these two signaling axes will further improve the treatment effects for patients with renal diseases.

3. Conclusions

As our understanding of the RAAS system deepens, there is potential for the development of more targeted drugs with fewer side effects. For instance, medications targeting the ACE2/Ang-(1–7)/Mas axis may aid in the treatment of hypertension and diabetic nephropathy. Personalized treatment plans could also be provided based on a patient's genotype and phenotype. For example, the selection of the most appropriate medication could be based on the patient's RAAS gene polymorphisms. Combined therapies that utilize drugs targeting different axes of the RAAS might produce synergistic effects, enhancing therapeutic outcomes. An example of this is the combined use of ACE inhibitors or ARBs with ACE2 agonists.

Despite current advancements in RAAS system research, the long-term use of RAAS inhibitors may lead to the development of tolerance in patients, and certain drugs may cause side effects such as coughing and hyperkalemia. Additionally, there are variations in patient responses to RAAS inhibitors that require further research to elucidate the causes of this heterogeneity. The high cost of new drug development poses a significant challenge in balancing the efficacy, safety, and economic cost of medications. Particularly, the interactions among the various components within the RAAS system are highly complex, making it difficult for a single drug to regulate the entire system comprehensively.

In summary, research and development of therapeutic strategies for the RAAS system is a field replete with challenges and opportunities. Future research needs to build upon a profound understanding of the RAAS system to develop novel treatment methods while addressing the limitations of existing therapeutic approaches. Through interdisciplinary collaboration, personalized medicine, and consideration of social ethics, more effective and safer treatment options can be provided for patients.

Acknowledgements

This paper was supported by the National Natural Science Foundation of China (No. 81760046) and Guizhou Provincial Natural Science Foundation (QKH [2018] 2758, QKH [2020]1Z058). The authors acknowledge the use of ChatGPT for language polishing of the manuscript.

Conflict of interest

The authors declare no conflict of interest.

Author details

Yan Qing Gong[1], Hao Liu[2], Zi Ce Su[1], Ming Chuan Ba[3], Xiao Min Li[3], Li Jun Li[3] and Hong Zhe Zhang[3]*

1 The Second Clinical Medical School, Southern Medical University, Guangzhou, China

2 The First School of Clinical Medicine, Jinan University, Guangzhou, China

3 The Seventh Affiliated Hospital of Southern Medical University, Foshan, China

*Address all correspondence to: zhz2593620@smu.edu.cn

References

[1] Stegbauer J, Oberhauser V, Vonend O, Rump LC. Angiotensin-(1-7) modulates vascular resistance and sympathetic neurotransmission in kidneys of spontaneously hypertensive rats. Cardiovascular Research. 2004;**61**(2):352-359

[2] Schmieder RE. Mechanisms for the clinical benefits of angiotensin II receptor blockers. American Journal of Hypertension. 2005;**18**(5):720-730

[3] RAS S, SVB P, Ferreira AJ. The ACE2-Ang-(1-7)-mas axis and cardioprotection. Current Cardiology Reviews. 2017;**3**(1):57-64

[4] Hellman N. Basic review: The renin-angiotensin-aldosterone axis [Internet]. Renal Fellow Network; 2009. p. 21. Available from: https://www.renalfellow.org/2009/08/28/basic-review-renin-angiotensin/ [Accessed: August 8, 2024]

[5] The Renin-Angiotensin-Aldosterone-System - TeachMePhysiology [Internet]. Available from: https://teachmephysiology.com/urinary-system/regulation/the-renin-angiotensin-aldosterone-system/ [Accessed: August 8, 2024]

[6] Circadian Clocks of the Kidney: Function, Mechanism, and Regulation - PubMed [Internet]. Available from: https://pubmed.ncbi.nlm.nih.gov/35575250/ [Accessed: July 23, 2024]

[7] Matsuyama T, Ohashi N, Aoki T, Ishigaki S, Isobe S, Sato T, et al. Circadian rhythm of the intrarenal renin-angiotensin system is caused by glomerular filtration of liver-derived angiotensinogen depending on glomerular capillary pressure in adriamycin nephropathy rats. Hypertension Research. 2021;**44**(6):618-627

[8] Pulakat L, Sumners C. Angiotensin type 2 receptors: Painful, or not? Frontiers in Pharmacology [Internet]. 2020;**11**:571994. DOI: 10.3389/fphar.2020.571994. Available from: https://www.sci-hub.ee/ [Accessed: August 8, 2024]

[9] Wu C, Liu H, Zha J, Gao Z, Li L, Xu P, et al. Angiotensin-converting enzyme - human amniotic mesenchymal stem cells improve pulmonary vascular remodeling in rats with pulmonary hypertension by promoting angiogenesis. International Journal of Clinical and Experimental Pathology. 2023;**16**(10):282-293

[10] Guo S, Wang^ D. Novel insights into the potential applications of stem cells in pulmonary hypertension therapy. Respiratory Research. 2024;**25**(1):237

[11] Madrigal Aguilar DA, Tufiño C, Fernandez-Martinez E, Bracho-Valdés I, Bobadilla Lugo RA. AT1R antagonism improves metabolic and vascular changes of obesity-induced gestational diabetes mellitus. Pathophysiology. 2019;**26**(2):121-127

[12] Urushihara M, Kagami S. Role of the intrarenal renin–angiotensin system in the progression of renal disease. Pediatric Nephrology. 2017;**32**(9):1471-1479

[13] Almeida LF, Tofteng SS, Madsen K, Jensen BL. Role of the renin-angiotensin system in kidney development and programming of adult blood pressure. Clinical Science London England 1979. 2020;**134**(6):641-656

[14] Frontiers. The ACE2/Angiotensin-(1-7)/Mas Receptor

Axis: Pleiotropic Roles in Cancer [Internet]. Available from: https://www.frontiersin.org/journals/physiology/articles/10.3389/fphys.2017.00276/full [Accessed: August 16, 2024]

[15] Shukla AK, Awasthi K, Usman K, Banerjee M. Role of renin-angiotensin system/angiotensin converting enzyme-2 mechanism and enhanced COVID-19 susceptibility in type 2 diabetes mellitus. World Journal of Diabetes. 2024;**15**(4):606-622

[16] Clinical Predictors of Accurate Prehospital Stroke Recognition - PubMed [Internet]. Available from: https://pubmed.ncbi.nlm.nih.gov/25922507/ [Accessed: August 12, 2024]

[17] Comparison of Methylprednisolone Plus Prednisolone with Prednisolone alone as Initial Treatment in Adult-Onset Minimal Change Disease: A Retrospective Cohort Study - PubMed [Internet]. Available from: https://pubmed.ncbi.nlm.nih.gov/24721890/ [Accessed: August 12, 2024]

[18] Discovery and *In vitro* and *In vivo* Profiles of N-ethyl-N-[2-[3-(5-fluoro-2-pyridinyl)-1H-pyrazol-1-yl]ethyl]-2-(2H-1,2,3-triazol-2-yl)-Benzamide as a Novel Class of Dual Orexin Receptor Antagonist - PubMed [Internet]. Available from: https://pubmed.ncbi.nlm.nih.gov/25693785/ [Accessed: August 12, 2024]

[19] Lim PO, MacFadyen RJ, Struthers AD. Is there a role for renin profiling in selecting chronic heart failure patients for ACE inhibitor treatment? Heart. 2000;**83**(3):257-261

[20] Dynamics of Anxiety in Women Undergoing Coronary Angiography - PubMed [Internet]. Available from: https://pubmed.ncbi.nlm.nih.gov/23990234/ [Accessed: August 12, 2024]

[21] Incidental Intraosseous Pneumatocyst with Gas-Density-Fluid Level in an Adolescent: A Case Report and Review of the Literature - PubMed [Internet]. Available from: https://pubmed.ncbi.nlm.nih.gov/24967024/ [Accessed: August 12, 2024]

[22] Kidney Cancer: Androgen Receptor—A New Target in Renal Cell Carcinoma? - PubMed [Internet]. Available from: https://pubmed.ncbi.nlm.nih.gov/24980195/ [Accessed: August 12, 2024]

[23] Berger S, Bleich M, Schmid W, Greger R, Schütz G. Mineralocorticoid receptor knockout mice: Lessons on Na^+ metabolism. Kidney International. 2000;**57**(4):1295-1298

[24] Zhu XF, Wang ZW, Wan JX, Sun Y, Wu YR, Li GX, et al. Pectin enhances rice (*Oryza sativa*) root phosphorus remobilization. Journal of Experimental Botany. Feb 2015;**66**(3):1017-1024. DOI: 10.1093/jxb/eru461. Epub 2014 Dec 20

[25] Simões SC, Balico-Silva AL, Parreiras-e-Silva LT, Bitencourt ALB, Bouvier M, Costa-Neto CM. Signal transduction profiling of angiotensin II type 1 receptor with mutations associated to atrial fibrillation in humans. Frontiers in Pharmacology [Internet]. 2020;**11**. Available from: https://www.frontiersin.org/journals/pharmacology/articles/10.3389/fphar.2020.600132/full [Accessed: August 12, 2024]

[26] Ciric I, Farhat H. The early versus late magnetic resonance imaging debate. World Neurosurgery. 2015;**83**(4):471-472

[27] Triple Dissociation of Duration Perception Regulating Mechanisms: Top-Down Attention is Inherent - PubMed [Internet]. Available from: https://://

pubmed.ncbi.nlm.nih.gov/28792544/ [Accessed: August 12, 2024]

[28] Treatment Advances in Locoregionally Advanced and Stage IVB/Recurrent Cervical Cancer: Can We Agree That More Is Not Always Better? - PubMed [Internet]. Available from: https://pubmed.ncbi.nlm.nih.gov/25987695/ [Accessed: August 12, 2024]

[29] Sparks MA, Dilmen E, Ralph DL, Rianto F, Hoang TA, Hollis A, et al. Vascular control of kidney epithelial transporters. The American Journal of Physiology-Renal Physiology. 2021;**320**(6):F1080-F1092

[30] The Angiotensin II Type 1(AT1) Receptor and Cardiac Hypertrophy: Did We Have It Wrong All Along? - PubMed [Internet]. Available from: https://pubmed.ncbi.nlm.nih.gov/33657051/ [Accessed: August 12, 2024]

[31] Poznyak AV, Bezsonov EE, Eid AH, Popkova TV, Nedosugova LV, Starodubova AV, et al. ACE2 is an adjacent element of atherosclerosis and COVID-19 pathogenesis. International Journal of Molecular Sciences. 2021;**22**(9):4691

[32] Wang SC, Wang YF. Cardiovascular protective properties of oxytocin against COVID-19. Life Sciences. 2021;**270**:119130

[33] Tajbakhsh A, Gheibi Hayat SM, Taghizadeh H, Akbari A, Inabadi M, Savardashtaki A, et al. COVID-19 and cardiac injury: Clinical manifestations, biomarkers, mechanisms, diagnosis, treatment, and follow up. Expert Review of Anti-Infective Therapy. 2021;**19**(3):345-357

[34] Kluck GEG, Yoo JA, Sakarya EH, Trigatti BL. Good cholesterol gone bad? HDL and COVID-19. International Journal of Molecular Sciences. 2021;**22**(19):10182

[35] Tang Y, Hu L, Liu Y, Zhou B, Qin X, Ye J, et al. Possible mechanisms of cholesterol elevation aggravating COVID-19. International Journal of Medical Sciences. 2021;**18**(15):3533-3543

[36] de Lelis DF, de Freitas DF, Machado AS, Crespo TS, SHS S. Angiotensin-(1-7), adipokines and inflammation. Metabolism. 2019;**95**:36-45

[37] Angiotensin-Converting Enzyme 2: SARS-CoV-2 Receptor and Regulator of the Renin-Angiotensin System: Celebrating the 20th Anniversary of the Discovery of ACE2 - PubMed [Internet]. Available from: https://pubmed.ncbi.nlm.nih.gov/32264791/ [Accessed: August 16, 2024]

[38] Patel VB, Parajuli N, Oudit GY. Role of angiotensin-converting enzyme 2 (ACE2) in diabetic cardiovascular complications. Clinical Science London England 1979. 2014;**126**(7):471-482

[39] Salih M, Bovée DM, van der Lubbe N, Danser AHJ, Zietse R, Feelders RA, et al. Increased urinary extracellular vesicle sodium transporters in cushing syndrome with hypertension. The Journal of Clinical Endocrinology and Metabolism. 2018;**103**(7):2583-2591

[40] Tenschert W, Baumgart P, Greminger P, Vetter W, Vetter H. Pathogenetic aspects of hypertension in Cushing's syndrome. Cardiology. 1985;**72**(Suppl. 1):84-90

[41] Liu C, Zheng F, Zhang X, Pan J, Ding W, Tian X. Selective venous sampling for secondary hypertension. Hypertension Research. 2024;**47**(7):1766-1778

[42] The Apelin-APJ System in the Evolution of Heart Failure - PubMed [Internet]. Available from: https://pubmed.ncbi.nlm.nih.gov/26528040/ [Accessed: August 16, 2024]

[43] The Role of Renin-Angiotensin-Aldosterone System in the Heart and Lung: Focus on COVID-19 - PubMed [Internet]. Available from: https://pubmed.ncbi.nlm.nih.gov/33959029/ [Accessed: August 16, 2024]

[44] Screening for Genetic Causes of Hypertension - PubMed [Internet]. Available from: https://pubmed.ncbi.nlm.nih.gov/12419172/ [Accessed: August 16, 2024]

[45] High Plasma Adrenomedullin Concentrations in Patients with High-Renin Essential Hypertension - PubMed [Internet]. Available from: https://pubmed.ncbi.nlm.nih.gov/12228854/ [Accessed: August 16, 2024]

[46] Role of Angiotensin-Converting Enzyme 2 (ACE2) in Diabetic Cardiovascular Complications - PubMed [Internet]. Available from: https://pubmed.ncbi.nlm.nih.gov/24329564/ [Accessed: August 16, 2024]

[47] Haase M, Dringenberg T, Allelein S, Willenberg HS, Schott M. Excessive catecholamine secretion and the activation of the renin-angiotensin-aldosterone-system in patients with pheochromocytoma: A single center experience and overview of the literature. Hormone and Metabolic Research. 2017;**49**(10):748-754

[48] Angiotensin-(1-7): A Novel Peptide to Treat Hypertension and Nephropathy in Diabetes? - PubMed [Internet]. Available from: https://pubmed.ncbi.nlm.nih.gov/26793405/ [Accessed: August 16, 2024]

[49] Homocysteine, Renin and Aldosterone in Patients With Cushing's Syndrome - PubMed [Internet]. Available from: https://pubmed.ncbi.nlm.nih.gov/18597007/ [Accessed: August 16, 2024]

[50] Advances in Understanding the Renin-Angiotensin-Aldosterone System (RAAS) in Blood Pressure Control and Recent Pivotal Trials of RAAS Blockade In Heart Failure and Diabetic Nephropathy - PubMed [Internet]. Available from: https://pubmed.ncbi.nlm.nih.gov/28413612/ [Accessed: August 16, 2024]

[51] Angiotensin IV Attenuates Diabetic Cardiomyopathy via Suppressing FoxO1-Induced Excessive Autophagy, Apoptosis and Fibrosis - PubMed [Internet]. Available from: https://pubmed.ncbi.nlm.nih.gov/34522203/ [Accessed: August 16, 2024]

[52] Clinical Efficacy of a Benazepril and Spironolactone Combination in Dogs With Congestive Heart Failure due to Myxomatous Mitral Valve Disease: The BEnazepril Spironolactone STudy (BESST) - PubMed [Internet]. Available from: https://pubmed.ncbi.nlm.nih.gov/34028078/ [Accessed: August 16, 2024]

[53] Epstein M, Reaven NL, Funk SE, McGaughey KJ, Oestreicher N, Knispel J. Evaluation of the treatment gap between clinical guidelines and the utilization of renin-angiotensin-aldosterone system inhibitors. The American Journal of Managed Care. 2015;**21**(Suppl. 11):S212-S220

[54] New Therapies for Hyperkalemia - PubMed [Internet]. Available from: https://pubmed.ncbi.nlm.nih.gov/30865167/ [Accessed: August 16, 2024]

[55] The Renin-Angiotensin-Aldosterone System: A Crossroad from Arterial Hypertension to Heart Failure - PubMed [Internet]. Available from: https://pubmed.ncbi.nlm.nih.gov/31512149/ [Accessed: August 16, 2024]

[56] A Protective Erythropoietin Evolutionary Landscape, NLRP3 Inflammasome Regulation, and Multisystem Inflammatory Syndrome in Children - PubMed [Internet]. Available from: https://pubmed.ncbi.nlm.nih.gov/36310304/ [Accessed: August 16, 2024]

[57] Angioedema Induced by Cardiovascular Drugs: New Players Join Old Friends - PubMed [Internet]. Available from: https://pubmed.ncbi.nlm.nih.gov/26119220/ [Accessed: August 16, 2024]

[58] Neurohormonal Modulation as a Therapeutic Target in Pulmonary Hypertension - PubMed [Internet]. Available from: https://pubmed.ncbi.nlm.nih.gov/33266371/ [Accessed: August 16, 2024]

[59] Paulis L, Unger T. Novel therapeutic targets for hypertension. Nature Reviews. Cardiology. 2010;**7**(8):431-441

[60] Stanek A, Brożyna-Tkaczyk K, Myśliński W. The role of obesity-induced perivascular adipose tissue (PVAT) dysfunction in vascular homeostasis. Nutrients. 2021;**13**(11):3843

Chapter 3

Overview of Renin, Prorenin, and the Role of (Pro)Renin Receptor across the Organs and Potential Therapeutic Target

Lana Kourieh and Ola Arab

Abstract

The term renin can relate to either renin and prorenin enzymes. Both of these have been established to have a vital role in physiology, especially after discovering the (pro) renin receptor ((P)RR) that can bind to and activate both enzymes. Since binding to this receptor by renin/prorenin leads to angiotensin production and intracellular signaling cascades, (P)RR exhibits crucial roles in both physiological and pathophysiological processes across various organs including the kidneys, heart, and brain. Also, a cleaved form of (P)RR, known as soluble (pro)renin receptor (s(P)RR), has been identified. Current evidence suggests that both (P)RR and s(P)RR are crucial for the normal development and maintenance of vital organs. Dysfunction in these receptors is associated with diseases characterized by disrupted physiological homeostasis. This highlights the potential of (P)RR and s(P)RR as promising diagnostic and therapeutic targets.

Keywords: renin, prorenin, (pro)renin receptor, renin–angiotensin system, physiological, pathophysiological, therapeutic target

1. Introduction

The discovery of a specific receptor for renin and its precursor, prorenin, has changed our understanding of renin as merely an enzyme that cleaves angiotensinogen (AGT) and prorenin as just an "inactive" proenzyme. This receptor, known as (pro)renin receptor ((P)RR), binds renin and prorenin. When these enzymes attach to the receptor, their activity on the cell surface is enhanced, initiating intracellular signaling that modifies gene expression. This indicates that renin can also function as a hormone and that prorenin has a specific role [1].

Recent findings suggest that (P)RR plays a role in organ damage by contributing to high blood pressure, insulin resistance, fibrosis, cardiac remodeling, and cancer. Interestingly, blocking the interaction between prorenin and (P)RR with a potential blocker known as "handle region peptide" (HRP) has been reported to improve glucose tolerance and enhance insulin sensitivity. Additionally, a monoclonal antibody targeting the extracellular domain of (P)RR has been tested on human colorectal cancer cells. If these findings are accurate, (P)RR could become a significant therapeutic target [1, 2].

In 2009, researchers identified a 28-kDa soluble (pro)renin receptor (s(P)RR) in plasma [3]. This cleaved form of the full-length (P)RR can activate the renin-angiotensin system (RAS) independently of the full-length receptor, influencing physiological and pathophysiological processes through different mechanisms. The s(P)RR hormone, as part of the RAS, has been recognized as a plasma biomarker for hypertension and cardiovascular diseases in humans [4].

2. Renin and prorenin

2.1 Renin

Renin, which is also known as the active renin, is an aspartyl protease that consists of two main lobes with a split in between containing two aspartic residues, where the active site is localized. AGT is the only recognized substrate for renin. Renin splits AGT to produce angiotensin I (Ang I) which is later transformed into Ang II via the angiotensin-converting enzyme. Not only renin is substrate specific to AGT, it is also a species-specific enzyme; meaning that it is only active on AGT of the same species. Juxtaglomular apparatus (JGA) is the location of renin producing cells and the secretory granules where renin is stored in and released from after acute stimulation of the JGA [5].

Mainly renin is released into bloodstream in conditions that result in lower renal perfusion and decreased tubular sodium content, and its activity half-life in plasma is up to 15 minutes [6]. Triggering of renin release happens through four main stimuli [7–9]:

- Different levels of renal perfusion stimulate the pressure transducer mechanism in afferent arterioles.
- Levels of NaCl in the distal convoluted tubule which are detected by the JGA chemoreceptors.
- Increased stimulation of beta-1 adrenergic receptors.
- Low levels of angiotensin I, arterial natriuretic peptide (ANP), and potassium (negative feedback).

2.2 Prorenin

As the precursor of renin, prorenin is also identified as the inactive renin. Nevertheless, prorenin is equal to 70–90% of total renin in human plasma. The reason of enzymatic inactivity of prorenin is due to a pro-segment of 43-amino acid N-terminal that covers the split of the active site [5]. Unlike renin, prorenin is not exclusively synthesized in the JGA but also in many other tissues such as the Müller cells in the eye, the collecting duct, adrenal zona glomerulosa, mast cells, thecal cells in the ovary, myometrium and decidual cells in the uterus, chorionic cells in the placenta, Leydig cells in the testis, and submandibular gland [10]. Under normal circumstances, prorenin levels in plasma are 10 times of renin levels [11]. A recent study using a polyclonal antibody specified to the N-terminal of the pro-segment reported prorenin plasma levels in healthy human of 3–13.4 μg/mL, which are 100–1000 times higher than previous reports [12].

2.2.1 Activation of prorenin

While other proenzymes are autoactivated in the plasma such as trypsin, prorenin activation takes place under two conditions (**Figure 1**).

- *Proteolytic activation*: This activation is irreversible and happens in-vivo through the removal of the pro-segment by activation protease enzymes such as proconvertase 1 and cathepsin B leading to the active renin form. This process takes place in the renin producing cells of the JGA [5, 13, 14].

- *Non-proteolytic activation*: A reversible in vitro process happens by applying low pH (<0.3) which is called acid activation or low temperature (4°C) which is known as cryoactivation. Those methods, respectively, lead to complete activation and partial activation of prorenin. Non-proteolytic activation can be basically assumed as unfolding of the pro-segment away from the active site split leading to the open active form of prorenin. Approximately only 2% of prorenin is in the open, active form in the plasma (physiological conditions) [5, 14–17].

2.3 The (pro)renin receptor ((P)RR)

(P)RR is a single transmembrane protein receptor that consists of 350 amino acids with the N-terminal on the extracellular side, encoded on the X chromosome by the ATP6AP2 gene and was first cloned in 2002. The extracellular domain is large and can be cleaved to give a s(P)RR (**Figure 2**) [19, 20]. The cleavage takes place in the trans-Golgi by recognizing a specific amino acid sequence $R^{275}KTR^{278}$, hence giving a 10-kd cytoplasmic/transmembrane fragment (M8.9) that is associated with V-ATPase and a 28-kd domain secreted extracellularly, which represents the s(P)RR (**Figure 3**) [20]. The (P)RR cleavage has been first reported to happen by furin. However, a later study published that s(P)RR production is increased by a disintegrin and metalloproteinase 19 (ADAM19) and does not decrease by furin inhibition [3, 21]. Two more recent studies established the necessity of site-1-protease S1P for s(P)RR production upon recognition of amino acid sequence $R^{278}TIL^{281}$ [22, 23].

Both prorenin and renin bind to (P)RR, with renin having less affinity to bind to this receptor than prorenin [24]. When it binds to (P)RR, renin goes through a configuration change, which allows the substrate AGT to attach. Through this attachment, renin catalytic efficiency is increased by four-fold to turn AGT to Ang I [19].

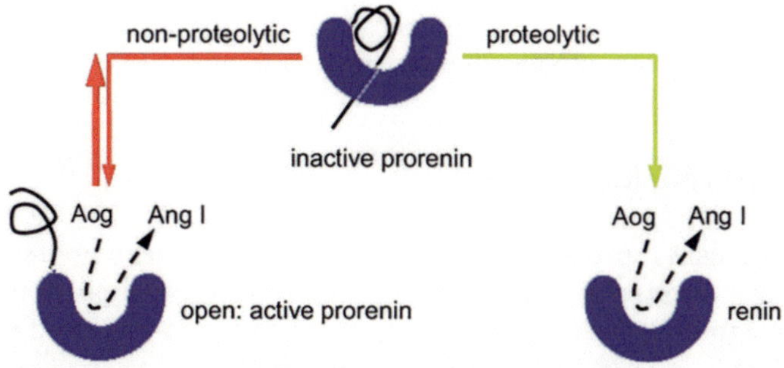

Figure 1.
Proteolytic and non-proteolytic activation of prorenin.

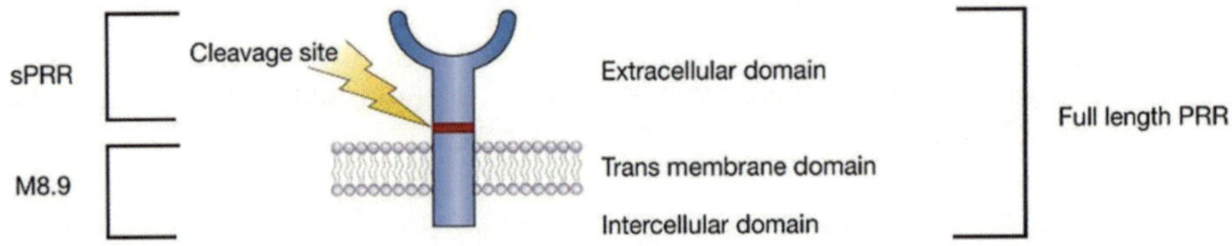

Figure 2.
Simplified illustration of the prorenin\renin receptor [18].

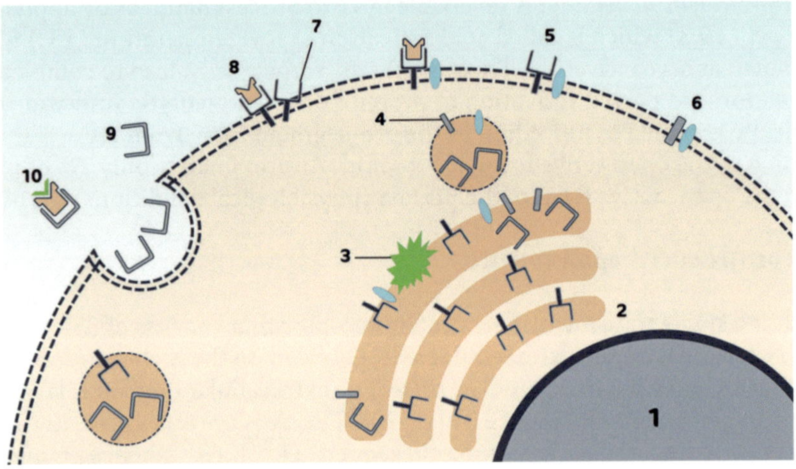

Figure 3.
(P)RR before and after cleavage. 1: nucleus, 2: trans golgi, 3: cleavage enzyme, 4: cytoplasmic domain of PRR, 5: V-ATPase complexed to full length PRR, 6: V-ATPase complexed to truncated length PRR/M8.9, 7: full length PRR, 8: renin, 9: soluble PRR, 10: PRO-renin.

As a matter of a fact, prorenin activation is possible when binding to this receptor as prorenin goes through configurational change at the pro-segment part, and hence, the active site is exposed and available for the substrate (nonproteolytic activation) [19, 25, 26].

Besides the renal glomeruli arteries, (P)RR has been detected in many tissues, such as the sub-endothelium of coronary arteries, the pituitary gland, the placenta, and the frontal lobes in the brain [27].

Recent studies indicate that similar to full length (P)RR, s(P)RR plays an important role in multiple physiopathologic processes, including tissue RAS activation [28] kidney injury [29], water balance regulation [30], and disease progress such as hypertension [31].

2.4 Renin/prorenin binding to (P)RR

Besides angiotensin II production, the (P)RR exhibits other angiotensin II independent functions (**Figure 4**). The binding of renin/prorenin to the (P)RR initiates an intracellular signaling pathway and activates the mitogen-activated protein (MAP) kinases ERK1/ERK2 and p38-heat shock protein, which leads to an upregulation of collagen, fibronectin (FN), transforming growth factor Beta 1 (TGFβ1), cyclo-oxygenase-2, and plasminogen activator inhibitor 1 (PAI1) [32–36]. Another worth

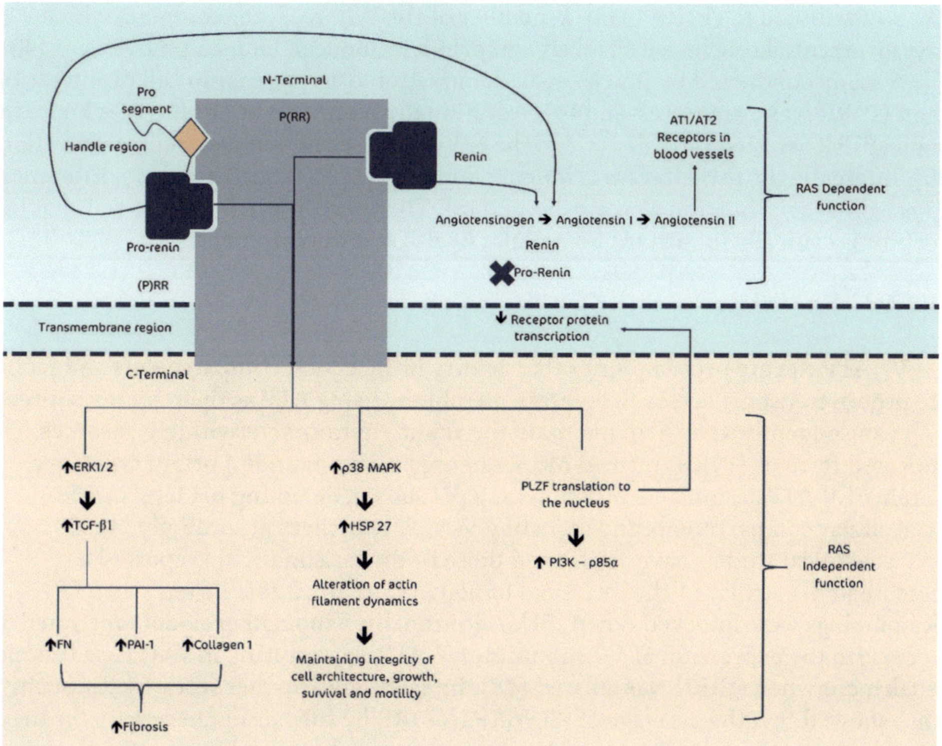

Figure 4.
Consequences of renin/prorenin binding to (P)RR.

mentioning pathway triggered by this binding is the phosphatidylinositol 3-kinase (PI3K-p85) pathway, which leads to nuclear translocation of the promyelocytic zinc finger transcription factor that is responsible for downregulation of the expression of (P)RR, meaning that high levels of renin/prorenin have a negative feedback effect on (P)RR expression, hence avoiding over activation [37, 38].

Irrelevant to renin/prorenin binding to (P)RR, the M8.9 domain is important for the vacuolar ATPase (V-ATPase) function which is involved in lysosomal acidification [39, 40]. (P)RR also functions as an adaptor between V-ATPase and low-density lipoprotein-related receptors 5 and 6 (LRP6/5), thereby activating the Wnt/β-catenin signaling pathway. This pathway plays a crucial role in metabolism, embryonic development, and cell differentiation [41]. Notably, this function is also exhibited by the s(P)RR [42].

3. (P)RR role in both physiological and pathophysiological processes across the organs

3.1 The physiological role of (P)RR

3.1.1 Cell cycle

Under normal conditions, a high concentration of (P)RR is found in the human heart, kidney, brain, and colon [42]. Numerous studies have confirmed the significant role of (P)RR in cell proliferation and cell cycle progression [43–45]. This crucial role may be attributed to (P)RR being a member of the Wnt receptor complex, which plays an essential role in cell survival and proliferation, cell fate, and movement [43–46]. A study conducted by Bracke et al. demonstrated an increase in cell proliferation when (P)RR was overexpressed [44]. Additionally, Wanka et al., found that knocking down (P)RR arrested the cell cycle in the G0/G1 phase and reduced cell proliferation [45]. Interestingly, this effect was independent of V-ATPase activity, as no differences in lysosomal acidification were observed [45]. Therefore, it can be concluded that this receptor is critically important for cellular health and development.

3.1.2 Acid-base balance

(V-)ATPases are proton pumps that acidify intracellular compartments and facilitate proton transport across the plasma membrane using ATP as their energy source [47]. Consequently, they help maintain the acidic environment within lysosomes. The truncated form of (P)RR, termed M8.9, not only serves as an important accessory protein of V-ATPase but also functions as a pH sensor, detecting pH levels within intracellular compartments and adjusting V-ATPase activity accordingly [48–50].

Two clinical studies have confirmed these findings. Zima et al., reported a decrease in the acidity of the intestinal lumen in *Caenorhabditis elegans* when (P)RR homologs were knocked down [51]. Additionally, Kinouchi et al. demonstrated a decrease in the expression of V0 subunits of V-ATPase, resulting in V-ATPase function impairment when (P)RR was ablated [48]. Interestingly, further study by Kinouchi et al., showed that the cleavage of ATP6AP2/(P)RR by furin is not necessary for the biogenesis of active V-ATPase, and M8.9 might simply be a residue after the cleavage of full-length (P)RR [49].

These results underscore the crucial role of (P)RR in maintaining the normal environment within lysosomes, and any disruption in its function can lead to cell death due to lysosomal acidification disorders.

3.1.3 Autophagy

Autophagy well known as a process where cells degrade and recycle their own components, which is essential for maintaining cellular health. This mechanism eliminates senescent cells and prevents the accumulation of damaged proteins, fats, and organelles, thus preserving protein quality and cellular balance. The rate of autophagy varies among different cell types; for instance, neurons exhibit higher autophagy levels compared to other cells [52]. Under normal physiological conditions, the body maintains a regulated rate of autophagy, which is crucial for protecting cellular function [53]. However, as people age, the rate of autophagy decreases, leading to the accumulation of damaged proteins. This decline contributes to the increased susceptibility of the elderly to heart attacks and neurological diseases [54, 55].

Autophagy is crucial during cellular nutrient deprivation or starvation, as it breaks down proteins and organelles to generate amino acids, replenishing nutrients and preventing cell death. Due to its vital role in cellular homeostasis, autophagy is tightly regulated [56]. Also, the regulation of autophagy is managed by the mammalian target of rapamycin (mTOR) pathway. Under nutrient-rich conditions, active mTOR inhibits autophagy. In contrast, during nutrient deprivation or stress, reduced mTOR activity initiates autophagy [56]. A regulatory network between mTOR and V-ATPase subunit expression has also been identified. In cells with abnormally high mTOR activity, V-ATPase subunit expression, including (P)RR/ATP6AP2, was increased.

This indicates mTOR regulates V-ATPase subunit expression, creating a positive feedback loop where V-ATPase subunits are essential for maintaining mTOR activity and vice versa (**Figure 5**) [57].

The addition of V-ATPase inhibitors to HEK293 cell cultures inhibited mTOR activity. Immunoprecipitation studies revealed interactions between V-ATPase subunits and the Rag-Regulator complex, crucial for forming the active mTOR signaling complex 1 (mTORC1). This suggests V-ATPase is vital for mTOR activity by sensing cellular nutrient states and modulating mTORC1 and Rag-Regulator interactions [50].

Autophagy was dysfunction in the hearts of mice with cardiomyocyte-specific (P)RR knockout [48], as well as in (P)RR-ablated cardiomyocytes, podocytes [58, 59], and vascular smooth muscle cells [60]. Specifically, loss of the V0 subunit of the V-ATPase due to (P)RR suppression leads to impaired autophagy. Consequently, (P)RR-dependent V-ATPase activity might affect autophagy by altering mTOR function. The impact of increased (P)RR expression on autophagy remains complex, as it could either enhance autophagic flux through vesicular acidification or suppress autophagy via mTOR signaling.

3.2 The pathophysiological role of (P)RR

3.2.1 Hypertension

High blood pressure (BP) is commonly associated with (P)RR, which influences BP through its effects on various organs.

3.2.1.1 The brain

(P)RR is primarily expressed in neurons within key cardiovascular regulatory areas in the brain, including the subfornical organ (SFO), paraventricular nucleus (PVN), rostral ventral lateral medulla (RVLM), nucleus tractus solitarii (NTS), and area postrema (AP) [61]. (P)RR is also found in astrocytes of the lateral cortex [62] and hypothalamic microglia, where its activation can lead to the release of pro-inflammatory cytokines through the NF-κB pathway [61]. In the supraoptic nucleus (SON) and subfornical organ (SFO), (P)RR appears to be prohypertensive [61, 63], as Shan et al. showed that reducing (P)RR expression in the SON of spontaneously

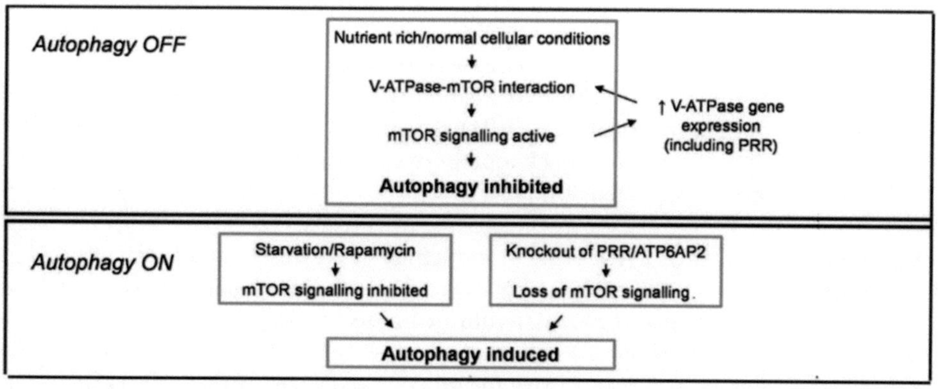

Figure 5.
Diagram of autophagy regulation mechanisms.

hypertensive rats (SHRs) lowered BP and heart rate [63]. Similarly, (P)RR knockdown in the SFO of hypertensive mice reduced BP and improved baroreceptor reflex sensitivity [61]. Conversely, in the nucleus tractus solitarii (NTS), (P)RR has an antihypertensive role, as Zubcevic et al., demonstrated that (P)RR knockdown in the NTS increased mean arterial pressure [64].

Also, Shan et al., showed that (P)RR overexpression stimulated vasopressin (AVP) secretion in normotensive rats without affecting BP [63]. (P)RR's ability to facilitate Ang II generation was confirmed by co-incubation studies. Further research demonstrated that (P)RR knockdown decreased BP and angiotensin II type 1 receptor (AT1R) and AVP levels in Ang II-dependent hypertensive mice [61, 65]. (P)RR knockout in salt-sensitive hypertensive mice prevented brain Ang II generation, highlighting (P)RR's role in brain RAS regulation and water balance via AVP [66]. Villar-Cheda et al., found that Ang II treatment increased (P)RR mRNA expression in dopaminergic neurons, reversible by losartan, suggesting (P)RR's role in Ang II-dependent hypertension [67].

The autonomic nervous system, particularly central sympathetic activity, plays a crucial role in raising BP. Studies have shown that (P)RR influences BP by increasing NADPH oxidase (NOX) 2 and NOX4 mRNA levels via the MAPK/ERK1/2 pathway, leading to reactive oxygen species (ROS) production [68] and the NOD-like receptor family pyrin domain containing 3 (NLRP3) inflammasomes activation [69]. These mechanisms highlight (P)RR's role in BP regulation, offering new avenues for treating neurological hypertension.

3.2.1.2 The kidney

Kidney plays a crucial role in BP regulation, with (P)RR being a significant factor. (P)RR enhances the activation of the local RAS in the renal medulla and collecting duct [70, 71], which is essential for managing extracellular fluid volume and salt reabsorption. Additionally, (P)RR impacts kidney function and BP through several other mechanisms:

- *Cyclooxygenase 2 (COX2) interaction*: COX2 as a key enzyme in prostaglandin production is a significant therapeutic target and increases renin activity in the kidney [72, 73]. Gonzalez et al., have indicated that (P)RR enhances COX2 expression independently of Ang II in rat renal medullary cells via ERK1/2 activation [74]. Also, (P)RR and COX2 expression both increase in the renal medulla, contributing to BP elevation in Ang II-dependent hypertensive mice. COX2 inhibitors can partially reduce BP in these cases [75]. Some studies suggest that COX2 elevates (P)RR expression through its product prostaglandin E2 (PGE2), with the e-prostanoid 4 (EP4) receptor playing a crucial role [76, 77]. This indicates a positive feedback loop between (P)RR and COX2, important in Ang II-dependent hypertension [78].

- *Sodium reabsorption*: (P)RR's role in inducing the expression and activation of α-epithelial sodium channels (α-ENaC) and other ion transporters is critical for sodium reabsorption and vascular volume homeostasis [79].

- *V-ATPase function*: As an accessory protein of V-ATPase, (P)RR affects the acidification of intracellular compartments, which is vital for various cellular processes, including ion transporter function. Its absence severely impairs

V-ATPase function, leading to the downregulation of important ion transporters, renal concentration defects, and distal renal tubular acidosis [48, 80].

- *Aquaporin-2 (AQP2) regulation*: (P)RR might influence water retention and urine concentration through AQP2 activation [81], which is a water channel regulated by vasopressin, and govern the water permeability of the luminal membrane in the collecting duct [82].

These mechanisms collectively highlight (P)RR's multifaceted role in kidney function and BP regulation. It is a complex but fascinating interplay that underscores the importance of (P)RR in maintaining overall health.

3.2.2 Fibrosis

Fibrosis is characterized by the excessive growth, hardening, and scarring of tissues due to the accumulation of extracellular matrix (ECM) components like collagen and fibronectin (FN). This excessive buildup, often triggered by chronic inflammatory reactions from various stimuli such as persistent infections, autoimmune responses, allergic reactions, chemical exposures, radiation, and tissue injury, can lead to organ dysfunction in the heart, lungs, liver, kidneys, and more [83, 84].

(P)RR plays a significant role in fibrosis through various pathways, independent of prorenin. In research done by He et al. (P)RR signaling was shown to stimulate cell proliferation and increases the buildup of type IV collagen and TGFβ1 expression via the ERK pathways in mesangial cells [85]. Also in heart, Ichihara et al., demonstrated that nonproteolytic activation of prorenin in tissue RAS leading to cardiac fibrosis in genetic hypertension [86]. (P)RR's involvement extends to several other organs, such as vascular smooth muscle cells [25], lungs [87], and eyes [88]. It also activates Wnt/β-catenin signaling, contributing to renal fibrosis, with elevated (P)RR expression observed in chronic kidney disease and related conditions [89]. Interestingly, (P)RR's activation of Wnt/β-catenin occurs independently of prorenin [89]. However, prorenin can enhance (P)RR expression and related fibrosis markers in renal tubular cells, suggesting a complex interplay between (P)RR, prorenin, and fibrosis pathways [90]. While the exact mechanisms are not fully understood, (P)RR appears to play a multifaceted role in promoting fibrosis under certain conditions. This highlights the need for further research to fully elucidate (P)RR's functions and potential as a therapeutic target in fibrotic diseases.

3.2.3 Cardiovascular disease (CVD)

(P)RR plays a role in cardiac remodeling, a process involving cardiomyocyte hypertrophy, apoptosis, and fibrosis, influenced by both RAS-dependent and independent pathways [91]. Increased (P)RR expression has been observed post-myocardial infarction and in conditions like dilated cardiomyopathy [92]. Studies suggest that (P)RR activation, through various mechanisms, contributes to cardiac remodeling and heart failure pathophysiology [93–95].

In 2012, research found that (P)RR blockade using HRP in sheep with heart failure decreased atrial pressure and Ang II levels, improving renal function [93]. Another study done by Yoshida et al., demonstrated that (P)RR blockade reduced fibrosis and hypertrophy by decreasing ERK1/2 activation and TGF-β expression, without affecting autophagy [94]. Recent studies by Zhang et al., demonstrated that (P)RR decoy inhibitor, PRO20, effectively reduces ROS generation and endoplasmic reticulum

(ER) stress, increasing cAMP levels and mitigating cardiac remodeling in heart failure [95]. These findings highlight the potential therapeutic benefits of PRO20 in addressing cardiac remodeling and related conditions. However, gene silencing of (P)RR in mice with heart failure induced by transverse aortic constriction (TAC) surgery led to autophagic flux blockade, causing an imbalance in ROS production and cardiac dysfunction [96]. Despite this, the therapeutic effects of (P)RR blockade in heart failure are significant, indicating a need to block (P)RR function without decreasing its gene expression. Additionally, two studies explore the role of the (P)RR in myocardial ischemia/reperfusion injury (IRI) by examining its effects on apoptosis and autophagy. Using a hypoxia/reoxygenation model in H9c2 cells, the researches investigate (P)RR-mediated pathways through both the p38 MAPK and β-catenin signaling pathways. The first study done by Liu et al., reveals that (P)RR activation significantly contributes to apoptosis via the p38 MAPK/caspase 3 pathway, independent of angiotensin II [97]. As for the second study by GAO et al., showed that (P)RR overexpression increases autophagy and promotes β-catenin pathway activity, which exacerbates cell death during IRI [98]. These findings highlight (P)RR as a potential therapeutic target for preventing myocardial IRI. Further in vivo studies are necessary to validate these results and explore (P)RR's therapeutic potential in clinical settings.

3.2.4 Lipid metabolism and atherosclerosis

Atherosclerosis, also known as coronary artery disease (CAD), is the most prevalent form of CVD. It primarily involves the accumulation of lipids and inflammation in the large arteries, which can ultimately lead to serious clinical complications such as myocardial infarction (MI) and stroke [99]. The disease's pathogenesis involves lipid metabolism disorders, with lipid deposition and lipid-phagocytosed macrophage accumulation playing vital roles in plaque formation [100]. Clinical evidence strongly associates dyslipidemia with atherosclerosis risk, particularly low-density lipoprotein (LDL), an independent predictor of CVD [101]. Recent studies suggest that the (P)RR is a component of lipid metabolism pathways, potentially contributing to atherosclerosis [102, 103]. (P)RR gene silencing reduces sortilin (SORT) 1 and LDL receptor abundance, impairing LDL uptake [102]. Additionally, (P)RR inhibition lowers plasma LDL-C and triglycerides, improving diet-induced obesity and liver steatosis by reducing lipid synthesis enzymes acetyl-CoA carboxylase (ACC) and pyruvate dehydrogenase (PDH) [104].

Atherosclerosis and vascular remodeling involve key events such as the migration and proliferation of vascular smooth muscle cells (VSMCs). (P)RR plays a crucial role in these processes. Studies have shown that prorenin binds to (P)RR in smooth muscle cells, promoting VSMC migration and proliferation by regulating plasminogen activator inhibitor-1 (PAI-1) expression [25, 105]. Further research identified prorenin as a chemotactic factor that, when combined with (P)RR, activates RhoA-GTP and Rac1-GTP, leading to cytoskeleton reorganization and VSMC migration [106]. Despite some conflicting evidence regarding the required concentration of prorenin, recent studies found that (P)RR overexpression facilitated Ang II-induced abdominal aortic aneurysm formation in apolipoprotein E-knockout mice [107]. This indicates that (P)RR can be activated by prorenin, renin, Ang II, or other factors.

In conclusion, (P)RR represents a promising therapeutic target for managing atherosclerosis and vascular remodeling. However, given the mixed findings and the intricate nature of its activation mechanisms, further research is essential to elucidate (P)RR's full range of actions and develop effective therapeutic strategies. The potential to modulate (P)RR activity to treat vascular diseases could lead to significant advancements in cardiovascular health.

3.2.5 Diabetic nephropathy

A study by Li et al., reported that in cultured podocytes, high glucose levels increase mRNA and protein (P)RR levels which clearly suggests that hyperglycemia in diabetic patients is related to (P)RR upregulation in podocytes, and hence, prorenin is also increased [108].

Under conditions of sustained hyperglycemia, in injured podocytes lysosomes and autophagosomes are formed in order to degrade degenerated proteins, which requires V-ATPase that is necessary for intracellular vesicles acidification. As mentioned before V-ATPase overexpress is correlated with (P)RR expression which is essential for V-ATPase activation. High prorenin levels in these diabetic patients binds to (P)RR resulting in RAS system enhancement and (P)RR-mediated mitogen-activated protein kinase signals expression, increasing harmful molecules involved in diabetic nephropathy progression such as COX2, interleukin-1β (IL-1β), TGFβ1, and tumor necrosis factor-α (TNF-α) [109].

3.2.6 Diabetic mellitus/glucose intolerance pathogenesis

As the stimulation of MAPK and TGFβ1-dependent pathways is induced by insulin, these pathways are assumed to have a contribution in the pathogenesis of insulin resistance [110, 111]. Also, MAPK p38 cascade is considered to have a role in β-cell function regulation. All together with the data of (P)RR-dependent stimulation of the mentioned intracellular pathways, it can be assumed that (P)RR may also contribute to the pathogenesis of glucose intolerance [112–115].

A specific type of V-ATPase, known as the a3 isoform, has been identified to play a role in the release of insulin from pancreatic β-cells [116]. In 3T3-F442A adipocytes, V-ATPase was shown to be engaged in insulin stimulated glucose transport [117]. Considering the connection between (P)RR and V-ATPase activation, it suggests another significant role of (P)RR in glucose intolerance, highlighting its diverse contributions to diabetes development [115]. Furthermore, there are indications from other studies suggesting an increase in renal medullary (P)RR expression in insulin resistance. Regarding gestational diabetes mellitus (GDM), a recent study suggested a potential link between elevated plasma levels of s(P)RR in pregnant women during the first trimester and the onset of GDM later in the third trimester [118].

3.2.7 Cancer

As mentioned earlier, (P)RR is expressed in various organs, including the brain, heart, liver, pancreas, placenta, and kidney. Beyond its role in enhancing the RAS, studies have confirmed that (P)RR is involved in numerous physiological and pathological processes, such as V-ATPase function, the MAPK/ERK pathway, and the Wnt/β-catenin signaling pathway. Recent research indicates that these pathways contribute to cancer initiation and progression, highlighting (P)RR's significant involvement.

Several studies demonstrated significantly an increase in (P)RR expression in cancers such as colorectal cancer [119], pancreatic ductal adenocarcinoma (PDAC) [120], glioma [121], breast carcinoma [122], and aldosterone-producing adenoma

[123], compared to normal tissues. (P)RR induces oncogenesis via Wnt signaling in pancreatic [124], colorectal [119], and brain [121] cancers and promotes endometrial cancer [125] and glioblastoma [126] through RAS. V-ATPase present on cancer cell membranes facilitates growth and invasion by engaging pathways like mTOR and TGFβ. Notably, elevated expression of (P)RR is associated with increased cell proliferation in breast carcinoma [122] and correlates with a poorer prognosis in glioma [121]. Additionally, higher levels of s(P)RR are observed in patients with PDAC [124]. Both studies by Koushi et al., and Shibayama et al., confirmed that when (P)RR expression is silenced using small interfering RNA (siRNA), cancer cell proliferation is reduced due to the inhibition of the Wnt/β-catenin signaling pathway [121, 124]. These findings suggest that (P)RR serves as a valuable prognostic marker and holds promise as a therapeutic target in various cancers.

4. s(P)RR relation with BP and CVD

Recent studies have highlighted the role of s(P)RR in hypertension and heart failure. Clinical research by Morimoto et al., showed a positive correlation between serum s(P)RR and serum creatinine levels in essential hypertension patients, but no correlation with BP [127]. Wang et al., suggested that sphingosine-1-phosphate (S1P), a cleavage site of full-length (P)RR, plays a role in hypertension, as blocking S1P improved Ang II-induced hypertension by reducing ENaC and AQP2 activation in the kidney. This effect was reversed by administration of recombinant s(P)RR [128]. Other studies found that recombinant s(P)RR impaired baroreflex sensitivity and increased BP in high-fat-fed mice due to enhanced sympathetic outflow [31]. Ramkumar et al., used CRISPR-Cas9 to mutate the (P)RR cleavage site, resulting in undetectable plasma s(P)RR levels, which reduced BP and renal injury in Ang II-induced hypertensive mice [129]. Additionally, s(P)RR might directly bind and activate the AT1R, leading to increased BP and endothelial dysfunction in obesity-related hypertensive mice [130]. These findings suggest that s(P)RR is a potential diagnostic and therapeutic tool in hypertension.

Regarding heart failure, studies are limited but revealing. In 2020, a clinical study by Obradovic et al., showed elevated s(P)RR levels in heart failure patients, with higher levels associated with lower left ventricular ejection fractions and greater left ventricular dilation in elderly heart failure patients. Recent studies suggest that s(P)RR, by activating AT1R, might contribute to heart disease pathogenesis [131]. Some researchers propose that s(P)RR induces tissue fibrosis via the PI3K-AKT pathway and oxidative stress via NOX4 in renal cells, but its effects on the myocardium are still unclear [132]. Clinical research found a correlation between high plasma s(P)RR levels and left ventricular remodeling, especially in chronic heart failure patients with reduced ejection fraction and renal dysfunction [133]. These findings suggest that s(P)RR could be a biomarker for chronic heart failure severity, warranting further research.

5. The relation of (P)RR & s(P)RR with preeclampsia

The maternal circulating RAAS, placental RAS, and intrarenal renin-angiotensin system (iRAS) play crucial roles in maternal cardiovascular and renal adaptations during pregnancy [134–136]. Dysregulation of these systems can significantly impact maternal and fetal health, leading to hypertensive disorders such as preeclampsia. Preeclampsia, a severe form of pregnancy-induced hypertension, involves widespread vascular endothelial dysfunction and can result in maternal and/or fetal death [137]. Elevated levels of (P)RR and s(P)RR are observed in preeclamptic pregnancies, potentially disrupting the regulation of RAS pathways and contributing to the pathogenesis of preeclampsia [138]. Interestingly, elevated s(P)RR during the first trimester predicts subsequent BP elevation [139] and increased rates of GDM [118], as mentioned before.

Despite no correlation existing between placental (P)RR expression and plasma s(P)RR levels, both are elevated in preeclampsia, indicating independent regulation [140]. Elevated (P)RR levels and oxidative stress in preeclamptic placentas enhance local RAS signaling [141]. Although RAS activity is increased, the functional implications in preeclampsia remain unclear, necessitating further research. Studies indicate elevated AT1R protein levels and increased renin expression in preeclamptic placentas [141, 142], emphasizing the need for more exploration to understand the roles of (P)RR and s(P)RR in preeclampsia.

Studies suggest that elevated levels of s(P)RR in preeclamptic pregnancies may contribute to the condition by impairing renal function and causing endothelial dysfunction, leading to hypertension [130, 140]. Despite variations in findings, Schofield et al., confirmed that increased levels of s(P)RR are associated with higher BP and reduced fetal growth [143]. Additionally, preeclamptic pregnancies show altered maternal circulating RAS components [144], including elevated prorenin levels [139] and enhanced (P)RR activity, which promote the formation of Ang I [145]. Elevated s(P)RR levels in preeclamptic patients can increase the activity of the circulating and iRAS. Despite reduced circulating levels of renin, ACE, Ang I, and Ang II, preeclampsia patients exhibit heightened sensitivity to Ang II/AT1R signaling, likely due to AT1R heterodimerization with the bradykinin receptor and elevated AT1R autoantibodies [144, 146, 147]. Enhanced s(P)RR/AT1R signaling may significantly increase AT1R activity, exacerbating hypertension and influencing maternal BP [138]. Understanding these mechanisms is essential for improving the management of preeclampsia.

Ang II signaling is crucial for iRAS activation. In vivo rat studies have shown that elevated intrarenal Ang II levels, resulting from AT1R-mediated uptake, stimulate iRAS, leading to increased intratubular Ang II production, distal sodium reabsorption, and renal damage [148, 149]. Additionally, elevated serum s(P)RR levels in preeclamptic pregnancies may enhance AT1R stimulation, similarly affecting iRAS [130]. In a 5/6 nephrectomy mouse model, increased urinary/renal levels of renin, AGT, and Ang II were observed [150]. Treatment with a (P)RR antagonist, PRO20, reduced these levels and impaired active-β-catenin in the renal cortex, indicating that (P)RR may mediate renal injuries through iRAS activation and/or β-catenin signaling, potentially contributing to renal injury in preeclampsia [150]. Understanding the mechanisms of s(P)RR in preeclampsia could improve diagnostic and therapeutic approaches for managing hypertensive disorders and renal injury during pregnancy.

6. Future perspectives: Applications in diagnosis and targeting

Given the close correlation between (P)RR expression levels in tumor tissues and the grades and stages of various cancers, (P)RR expression could serve as an adjunct marker alongside existing cancer-related protein markers. This combination could aid in diagnosis, assess disease severity, and predict prognosis for different cancers [151]. An s(P)RR ELISA kit has been developed to measure s(P)RR in blood and urine samples [152], revealing increased serum s(P)RR levels in patients with congestive heart failure (CHF) [153], kidney disease [154], hypertension [155], and preeclampsia [139]. These findings suggest that plasma s(P)RR could serve as a predictive biomarker not only in certain cancer contexts but also in several disorders.

Shibayama et al., demonstrated that plasma s(P)RR levels in patients with PDAC are significantly higher than in healthy controls [124]. Human PDAC cell lines also secreted much higher levels of s(P)RR compared to normal pancreatic epithelial cells, suggesting that plasma s(P)RR could serve as a promising predictive biomarker for PDAC. Additionally, Larrinaga et al., using tissue microarrays, suggested that PRR is a prognostic marker in invasive urothelial cancer of the bladder [156]. However, recent studies highlight that s(P)RR's predictive value in colorectal cancer (CRC) and primary epithelial ovarian cancer (EOC) is unclear. Maider et al. found no significant difference in s(P)RR levels between CRC patients and healthy controls [157], and Katrin et al. observed no correlation between s(P)RR levels and clinicopathological outcomes in EOC patients [158]. These findings suggest that s(P)RR is not a reliable predictive, prognostic, or diagnostic marker for EOC.

In a previous study, researchers developed a monoclonal antibody targeting the extracellular domain of (P)RR, specifically the amino acids 200 to 213. This antibody was tested on human colorectal cancer cells (DLD-1 and HCT116). The results demonstrated that the (P)RR antibody significantly inhibited cell proliferation compared to a negative control (human IgG). These findings indicate a promising potential for the (P)RR antibody as a therapy for colon cancer, and ongoing studies are further exploring its effectiveness [151].

Author details

Lana Kourieh* and Ola Arab
Department of Biochemistry and Microbiology, College of Pharmacy, Aleppo University, Aleppo, Syria

*Address all correspondence to: kouriehlana@gmail.com

References

[1] Nguyen G, Contrepas A. Renin, Prorenin, and the (pro) renin receptor. In: DeMello W, Frohlich E, editors. Renin Angiotensin System and Cardiovascular Disease, Contemporary Cardiology. 2nd ed. Paris, France: Humana Press; 2009. pp. 19-28. DOI: 10.1007/978-1-60761-186-8_3

[2] Ichihara A, Yatabe MS. The (pro)renin receptor in health and disease. Nature Reviews. Nephrology. 2019;**15**:693-712. DOI: 10.1038/s41581-019-0160-5

[3] Cousin C, Bracquart D, Contrepas A, Corvol P, Muller L, Nguyen G. Soluble form of the (pro)renin receptor generated by intracellular cleavage by furin is secreted in plasma. Hypertension. 2009;**53**(6):1077-1082. DOI: 10.1161/HYPERTENSIONAHA.108.127258

[4] Arthur G. Role of renal-derived human soluble prorenin receptor in blood pressure regulation and kidney function [thesis]. USA: University of Kentucky, Pharmacology and Nutritional Sciences; 2023. p. 53

[5] Danser AHJ, Deinum J. Renin, prorenin and the putative (pro) renin receptor. Hypertension. 2005;**46**:1069-1076. DOI: 10.1161/01.HYP.0000186329.92187.2e

[6] Skrabal F. Half-life of plasma renin activity in normal subjects and in malignant hypertension. Klinische Wochenschrift. 1974;**52**:1173-1174. DOI: 10.1007/BF01466736

[7] Schweda F, Friis U, Wagner C, Skott O, Kurtz A. Renin release. Physiology (Bethesda, Md.). 2007;**22**:310-319. DOI: 10.1152/physiol.00024.2007

[8] Kurtz A. Control of renin synthesis and secretion. American Journal of Hypertension. 2012;**25**:839-847. DOI: 10.1038/ajh.2011.246. Epub 2012 Jan 12

[9] Kurtz A. Renin release: Sites, mechanisms, and control. Annual Review of Physiology. 2011;**73**:377-399. DOI: 10.1146/annurev-physiol-012110-142238

[10] Krop M, Danser AH. Circulating versus tissue renin-angiotensin system: On the origin of (pro)renin. Current Hypertension Reports. 2008:**10**(2):112-118. DOI: 10.1007/s11906-008-0022-1

[11] Leckie BJ, Birnie G, Carachi R. Renin in Wilms' tumor: Prorenin as an indicator. The Journal of Clinical Endocrinology and Metabolism. 1994;**79**:1742-1746. DOI: 10.1210/jcem.79.6.7989481

[12] Fujimoto K, Kawamura S, Bando S, Kamata Y, Kodera Y, Shichiri M. Circulating prorenin: Its molecular forms and plasma concentrations. Hypertension Research. 2021;**44**:674-684. DOI: 10.1038/s41440-022-01033-9

[13] Reudelhuber TL, Ramla D, Chiu L, Mercure C, Seidah NG. Proteolytic processing of human prorenin in renal and non-renal tissues. Kidney International. 1994;**46**:1522-1524. DOI: 10.1038/ki.1994.435

[14] Neves FA, Duncan KG, Baxter JD. Cathepsin B is a prorenin processing enzyme. Hypertension. 1996;**27**:514-517. DOI: 10.1161/01.hyp.27.3.514

[15] Derkx FHM, Deinum J, Lipovski M, Verhaar M, Fischli W, Schalekamp MADH. Nonproteolytic

"activation" of prorenin by active site-directed renin inhibitors as demonstrated by renin-specific monoclonal antibody. Journal of Biological Chemistry. 1992;**267**:22837-22842

[16] Pitarresi TM, Rubattu S, Heinrikson R, Sealey JE. Reversible cryoactivation of recombinant human prorenin. The Journal of Biological Chemistry. 1992;**267**:11753-11759. DOI: 10.1016/S0021-9258(19)49762-7

[17] Suzuki F, Hayakawa M, Nakagawa T, Nasir UM, Ebihara A, Iwasawa A, et al. Human prorenin has "gate and handle" regions for its non-proteolytic activation. The Journal of Biological Chemistry. 2003;**278**:22217-22222. DOI: 10.1074/jbc.M302579200

[18] Ramkumar N, Kohan DE. The (pro)renin receptor: An emerging player in hypertension and metabolic syndrome. Kidney International. 2019;**95**(5):1041-1052. DOI: 10.1016/j.kint.2018.10.042

[19] Nguyen G, Delarue F, Burcklé C, Bouzhir L, Giller T, Sraer JD. Pivotal role of the renin/prorenin receptor in angiotensin II production and cellular responses to renin. The Journal of Clinical Investigation. 2002;**109**:1417-1427. DOI: 10.1172/JCI0214276

[20] Nguyen G, Muller DN. The biology of the (pro)renin receptor. Journal of the American Society of Nephrology. 2010;**21**(1):18-23. DOI: 10.1681/ASN.2009030300

[21] Yoshikawa A, Aizaki Y, Kusano K, Kishi F, Susumu T, Iida S, et al. The (pro)renin receptor is cleaved by ADAM19 in the Golgi leading to its secretion into extracellular space. Hypertension Research. 2011;**34**(5):599-605. DOI: 10.1038/hr.2010.284

[22] Fang H, Xu C, Lu A, Zou CJ, Xie S, Chen Y, et al. (Pro)renin receptor mediates albumin-induced cellular responses: Role of site-1 protease-derived soluble (pro)renin receptor in renal epithelial cells. American Journal of Physiology. Cell Physiology. 2017;**313**(6):C632-C643. DOI: 10.1152/ajpcell.00006.2017

[23] Nakagawa T, Suzuki-Nakagawa C, Watanabe A, Asami E, Matsumoto M, Nakano M, et al. Site-1 protease is required for the generation of soluble (pro)renin receptor. Journal of Biochemistry. 2017;**161**(4):369-379. DOI: 10.1093/jb/mvw080

[24] Nabi AH, Suzuki F. Biochemical properties of renin and prorenin binding to the (pro)renin receptor. Hypertension Research. 2010;**33**:91-97. DOI: 10.1038/hr.2009.201

[25] Zhang J, Noble NA, Border WA, Owens RT, Huang Y. Receptor-dependent prorenin activation and induction of PAI-1 expression in vascular smooth muscle cells. American Journal of Physiology. Endocrinology and Metabolism. 2008;**295**:E810-E819. DOI: 10.1152/ajpendo.90264.2008

[26] Nurun NA, Uddin MN, Nakagawa T, Iwata H, Ichihara A, Inagami T, et al. Role of 'handle' region of prorenin prosegment in the non-proteolytic activation of prorenin by binding to membrane anchored (pro)renin receptor. Frontiers in Bioscience. 2007;**12**:4810-4817. DOI: 10.2741/2429

[27] Gonzalez AA, Lara LS, Luffman C, Seth DM, Prieto MC. Soluble form of the (pro)renin receptor is augmented in the collecting duct and urine of chronic angiotensin II-dependent hypertensive rats. Hypertension. 2011;**57**:859-864. DOI: 10.1161/HYPERTENSIONAHA.110.167957

[28] Xie S, Su J, Lu A, Lai Y, Mo S, Pu M, et al. Soluble (pro)renin receptor

promotes the fibrotic response in renal proximal tubule epithelial cells in vitro via the Akt/β-catenin/snail signaling pathway. American Journal of Physiology. Renal Physiology. 2020;**319**(5):F941-F953. DOI: 10.1152/ajprenal.00197.2020

[29] Takahashi K, Hiraishi K, Hirose T, Kato I, Yamamoto H, Shoji I, et al. Expression of (pro) renin receptor in the human brain and pituitary, and co-localisation with arginine vasopressin and oxytocin in the hypothalamus. Journal of Neuroendocrinology. 2010;**22**:453-459. DOI: 10.1111/j.1365-2826.2010.01980.x

[30] Lu X, Wang F, Xu C, Soodvilai S, Peng K, Su J, et al. Soluble (pro)renin receptor via β-catenin enhances urine concentration capability as a target of liver X receptor. Proceedings of the National Academy of Sciences of the United States of America. 2016;**113**(13):E1898-E1906. DOI: 10.1073/pnas.1602397113

[31] Gatineau E, Gong MC, Yiannikouris F. Soluble prorenin receptor increases blood pressure in high fat-fed male mice. Hypertension. 2019;**74**(4):1014-1020. DOI: 10.1161/HYPERTENSIONAHA.119.12906

[32] Huang Y, Wongamorntham S, Kasting J, Mc-Quillan D, Owens RT, Yu L, et al. Renin increases mesangial cell transforming growth factor-beta1 and matrix proteins through receptor-mediated, angiotensin II-independent mechanisms. Kidney International. 2006;**69**:105-113. DOI: 10.1038/sj.ki.5000011

[33] Sakoda M, Ichihara A, Kaneshiro Y, Takemitsu T, Nakazato Y, Nabi AHMN, et al. (Pro-)renin receptor-mediated activation of mitogen-activated protein kinases in human vascular smooth muscle cells. Hypertension Research. 2007;**30**:1139-1146. DOI: 10.1291/hypres.30.1139

[34] Kaneshiro Y, Ichihara A, Takemitsu T, Sakoda M, Suzuki F, Nakagawa T, et al. Increased expression of cyclooxygenase-2 in the renal cortex of human prorenin receptor gene-transgenic rats. Kidney International. 2006;**70**:641-646. DOI: 10.1038/sj.ki.5001627

[35] Feldt S, Batenburg WW, Mazak I, Maschke U, Wellner M, Kvakan H, et al. Prorenin and renin-induced extracellular signal-regulated kinase 1/2 activation in monocytes is not blocked by aliskiren or the handle-region peptide. Hypertension. 2008;**51**(3):682-688. DOI: 10.1161/HYPERTENSIONAHA.107.101444

[36] Saris JJ, PA t' H, Garrelds IM, DHW D, den Dunnen JT, JMJ L, et al. Prorenin induces intracellular signaling in cardiomyocytes independently of angiotensin II. Hypertension. 2006;**48**:564-571. DOI: 10.1161/01.HYP.0000240064.19301.1b

[37] Schefe JH, Neumann C, Goebel M, Danser J, Kirsch S, Gust R, et al. Prorenin engages the (pro-)renin receptor like renin and both ligand activities are unopposed by aliskiren. Journal of Hypertension. 2008;**26**:1787-1794. DOI: 10.1097/HJH.0b013e3283060f2e

[38] Schefe JH, Menk M, Reinemund J, Effertz K, Hobbs RM, Pandolfi PP, et al. A novel signal transduction cascade involving direct physical interaction of the renin/prorenin receptor with the transcription factor promyelocytic zinc finger protein. Circulation Research. 2006;**99**:1355-1366. DOI: 10.1161/01.RES.0000251700.00994.0d

[39] Ludwig J, Kerscher S, Brandt U, Pfeiffer K, Getlawi F, Apps DK, et al.

Identification and characterization of a novel 9.2-kDa membrane sector-associated protein of vacuolar proton-ATPase from chromaffin granules. The Journal of Biological Chemistry. 1998;**273**(18):10939-10947. DOI: 10.1074/jbc.273.18.10939

[40] Lu X, Garrelds IM, Wagner CA, Danser AH, Meima ME. (Pro)renin receptor is required for prorenin-dependent and -independent regulation of vacuolar H(+)-ATPase activity in MDCK.C11 collecting duct cells. American Journal of Physiology. Renal Physiology. 2013;**305**(3):F417-F425. DOI: 10.1152/ajprenal.00037.2013

[41] Ahmed BA, Seda O, Lavoie JL. (Pro)renin receptor as a new drug target. Current Pharmaceutical Design. 2011;**17**(33):3611-3621. DOI: 10.2174/138161211798220963

[42] Fagerberg L, Hallström BM, Oksvold P, Kampf C, Djureinovic D, Odeberg J, et al. Analysis of the human tissue-specific expression by genome-wide integration of transcriptomics and antibody-based proteomics. Molecular & Cellular Proteomics. 2014;**13**(2):397-406. DOI: 10.1074/mcp.M113.035600

[43] Schafer ST, Han J, Pena M, von Bohlen Und Halbach O, Peters J, Gage FH. The Wnt adaptor protein ATP6AP2 regulates multiple stages of adult hippocampal neurogenesis. The Journal of Neuroscience. 2015;**35**(12):4983-4998. DOI: 10.1523/JNEUROSCI.4130-14.2015

[44] Bracke A, Schäfer S, von Bohlen Und Halbach V, Klempin F, Bente K, Bracke K, et al. ATP6AP2 over-expression causes morphological alterations in the hippocampus and in hippocampus-related behaviour. Brain Structure & Function. 2018;**223**:2287-2302. DOI: 10.1007/s00429-018-1633-1

[45] Wanka H, Lutze P, Staar D, Peters B, Morch A, Vogel L, et al. (Pro) renin receptor (ATP6AP2) depletion arrests As4.1 cells in the G0/G1 phase thereby increasing formation of primary cilia. Journal of Cellular and Molecular Medicine. 2017;**21**:1394-1410. DOI: 10.1111/jcmm.13069

[46] Moon RT, Kohn AD, De Ferrari GV, Kaykas A. WNT and beta-catenin signalling: Diseases and therapies. Nature Reviews. Genetics. 2004;**5**(9):691-701. DOI: 10.1038/nrg1427

[47] Forgac M. Vacuolar ATPases: Rotary proton pumps in physiology and pathophysiology. Nature Reviews. Molecular Cell Biology. 2007;**8**(11):917-929. DOI: 10.1038/nrm2272

[48] Kinouchi K, Ichihara A, Sano M, Sun-Wada GH, Wada Y, Kurauchi-Mito A, et al. The (pro)renin receptor/ATP6AP2 is essential for vacuolar H^+-ATPase assembly in murine cardiomyocytes. Circulation Research. 2010;**107**(1):30-34. DOI: 10.1161/CIRCRESAHA.110.224667

[49] Kinouchi K, Ichihara A, Sano M, Sun-Wada GH, Wada Y, Ochi H, et al. The role of individual domains and the significance of shedding of ATP6AP2/(pro)renin receptor in vacuolar H(+)-ATPase biogenesis. PLoS One. 2013;**8**(11):e78603. DOI: 10.1371/journal.pone.0078603

[50] Zoncu R, Bar-Peled L, Efeyan A, Wang S, Sancak Y, Sabatini DM. mTORC1 senses lysosomal amino acids through an inside-out mechanism that requires the vacuolar H(+)-ATPase. Science. 2011;**334**(6056):678-683. DOI: 10.1126/science.1207056

[51] Zima V, Šebková K, Šimečková K, Dvořák T, Saudek V, Kostrouchová M. Prorenin receptor homologue VHA-20

is critical for intestinal pH regulation, ion and water management and larval development in *C. elegans*. Folia Biologica (Praha). 2015;**61**(5):168-177

[52] Mizushima N, Levine B, Cuervo AM, Klionsky DJ. Autophagy fights disease through cellular self-digestion. Nature. 2008;**451**(7182):1069-1075. DOI: 10.1038/nature06639

[53] Klionsky DJ, Emr SD. Autophagy as a regulated pathway of cellular degradation. Science. 2000;**290**:1717-1721. DOI: 10.1126/science.290.5497.1717

[54] Gustafsson AB, Gottlieb RA. Autophagy in ischemic heart disease. Circulation Research. 2009;**104**:150-158. DOI: 10.1161/CIRCRESAHA.108.187427

[55] Hara T, Nakamura K, Matsui M, Yamamoto A, Nakahara Y, Suzuki-Migishima R, et al. Suppression of basal autophagy in neural cells causes neurodegenerative disease in mice. Nature. 2006;**441**(7095):885-889. DOI: 10.1038/nature04724

[56] Binger KJ, Muller DN. Autophagy and the (pro)renin receptor. Frontiers in Endocrinology (Lausanne). 2013;**4**:155. DOI: 10.3389/fendo.2013.00155

[57] Peña-Llopis S, Vega-Rubin-de-Celis S, Schwartz JC, Wolff NC, Tran TA, Zou L, et al. Regulation of TFEB and V-ATPases by mTORC1. The EMBO Journal. 2011;**30**(16):3242-3258. DOI: 10.1038/emboj.2011.257

[58] Oshima Y, Kinouchi K, Ichihara A, Sakoda M, Kurauchi-Mito A, Bokuda K, et al. Prorenin receptor is essential for normal podocyte structure and function. Journal of the American Society of Nephrology. 2011;**22**(12):2203-2212. DOI: 10.1681/ASN.2011020202

[59] Riediger F, Quack I, Qadri F, Hartleben B, Park JK, Potthoff SA, et al. Prorenin receptor is essential for podocyte autophagy and survival. Journal of the American Society of Nephrology. 2011;**22**(12):2193-2202. DOI: 10.1681/ASN.2011020200

[60] Kurauchi-Mito A, Ichihara A, Bokuda K, Sakoda M, Kinouchi K, Yaguchi T, et al. Significant roles of the (pro)renin receptor in integrity of vascular smooth muscle cells. Hypertension Research. 2014;**37**(9):830-835. DOI: 10.1038/hr.2014.92

[61] Li W, Peng H, Cao T, Sato R, McDaniels SJ, Kobori H, et al. Brain-targeted (pro)renin receptor knockdown attenuates angiotensin II-dependent hypertension. Hypertension. 2012;**59**(6):1188-1194. DOI: 10.1161/HYPERTENSIONAHA.111.190108

[62] Li W, Peng H, Seth DM, Feng Y. The prorenin and (pro)renin receptor: New players in the brain renin-angiotensin system? International Journal of Hypertension. 2012;**2012**:290635. DOI: 10.1155/2012/290635

[63] Shan Z, Shi P, Cuadra AE, Dong Y, Lamont GJ, Li Q, et al. Involvement of the brain (pro)renin receptor in cardiovascular homeostasis. Circulation Research. 2010;**107**(7):934-938. DOI: 10.1161/CIRCRESAHA.110.226977

[64] Zubcevic J, Jun JY, Lamont G, Murça TM, Shi P, Yuan W, et al. Nucleus of the solitary tract (pro)renin receptor-mediated antihypertensive effect involves nuclear factor-κB-cytokine signaling in the spontaneously hypertensive rat. Hypertension. 2013;**61**(3):622-627. DOI: 10.1161/HYPERTENSIONAHA.111.199836

[65] Souza LAC, Worker CJ, Li W, Trebak F, Watkins T, Gayban AJB, et al. (Pro)renin receptor knockdown in the paraventricular nucleus of the

hypothalamus attenuates hypertension development and AT_1 receptor-mediated calcium events. American Journal of Physiology. Heart and Circulatory Physiology. 2019;**316**(6):H1389-H1405. DOI: 10.1152/ajpheart.00780.2018

[66] Li W, Peng H, Mehaffey EP, Kimball CD, Grobe JL, van Gool JM, et al. Neuron-specific (pro)renin receptor knockout prevents the development of salt-sensitive hypertension. Hypertension. 2014;**63**(2):316-323. DOI: 10.1161/HYPERTENSIONAHA.113.02041

[67] Villar-Cheda B, Costa-Besada MA, Valenzuela R, Perez-Costas E, Melendez-Ferro M, Labandeira-Garcia JL. The intracellular angiotensin system buffers deleterious effects of the extracellular paracrine system. Cell Death & Disease. 2017;**8**(9):e3044. DOI: 10.1038/cddis.2017.439

[68] Peng H, Li W, Seth DM, Nair AR, Francis J, Feng Y. (Pro)renin receptor mediates both angiotensin II-dependent and -independent oxidative stress in neuronal cells. PLoS One. 2013;**8**(3):e58339. DOI: 10.1371/journal.pone.0058339

[69] Hu L, Zhang S, Ooi K, Wu X, Wu J, Cai J, et al. Microglia-derived NLRP3 activation mediates the pressor effect of prorenin in the rostral ventrolateral medulla of stress-induced hypertensive rats. Neuroscience Bulletin. 2020;**36**(5):475-492. DOI: 10.1007/s12264-020-00484-9

[70] Xu C, Fang H, Zhou L, Lu A, Yang T. High potassium promotes mutual interaction between (pro)renin receptor and the local renin-angiotensin-aldosterone system in rat inner medullary collecting duct cells. American Journal of Physiology. Cell Physiology. 2016;**311**(4):C686-C695. DOI: 10.1152/ajpcell.00128.2016

[71] Wang F, Lu X, Liu M, Feng Y, Zhou SF, Yang T. Renal medullary (pro)renin receptor contributes to angiotensin II-induced hypertension in rats via activation of the local renin-angiotensin system. BMC Medicine. 2015;**13**:278. DOI: 10.1186/s12916-015-0514-1

[72] Turini ME, DuBois RN. Cyclooxygenase-2: A therapeutic target. Annual Review of Medicine. 2002;**53**:35-57. DOI: 10.1146/annurev.med.53.082901.103952

[73] Cheng HF, Harris RC. Cyclooxygenases, the kidney, and hypertension. Hypertension. 2004;**43**(3):525-530. DOI: 10.1161/01.HYP.0000116221.27079.ea

[74] Gonzalez AA, Luffman C, Bourgeois CR, Vio CP, Prieto MC. Angiotensin II-independent upregulation of cyclooxygenase-2 by activation of the (pro)renin receptor in rat renal inner medullary cells. Hypertension. 2013;**61**(2):443-449. DOI: 10.1161/HYPERTENSIONAHA.112.196303

[75] Gonzalez AA, Green T, Luffman C, Bourgeois CR, Gabriel Navar L, Prieto MC. Renal medullary cyclooxygenase-2 and (pro)renin receptor expression during angiotensin II-dependent hypertension. American Journal of Physiology. Renal Physiology. 2014;**307**(8):F962-F970. DOI: 10.1152/ajprenal.00267.2014

[76] Wang F, Lu X, Peng K, Zhou L, Li C, Wang W, et al. COX-2 mediates angiotensin II-induced (pro)renin receptor expression in the rat renal medulla. American Journal of Physiology. Renal Physiology. 2014;**307**(1):F25-F32. DOI: 10.1152/ajprenal.00548.2013

[77] Wang F, Lu X, Peng K, Du Y, Zhou SF, Zhang A, et al. Prostaglandin E-prostanoid4 receptor mediates

angiotensin II-induced (pro) renin receptor expression in the rat renal medulla. Hypertension. 2014;**64**(2):369-377. DOI: 10.1161/ HYPERTENSIONAHA.114.03654

[78] Yang T. Crosstalk between (pro) renin receptor and COX-2 in the renal medulla during angiotensin II-induced hypertension. Current Opinion in Pharmacology. 2015;**21**:89-94. DOI: 10.1016/j.coph.2014.12.011

[79] Peng K, Lu X, Wang F, Nau A, Chen R, Zhou SF, et al. Collecting duct (pro)renin receptor targets ENaC to mediate angiotensin II-induced hypertension. American Journal of Physiology. Renal Physiology. 2017;**312**:245-253. DOI: 10.1152/ ajprenal.00178.2016

[80] Trepiccione F, Gerber SD, Grahammer F, López-Cayuqueo KI, Baudrie V, Păunescu TG, et al. Renal Atp6ap2/(pro)renin receptor is required for normal vacuolar H+-ATPase function but not for the renin-angiotensin system. Journal of the American Society of Nephrology. 2016;**27**(11):3320-3330. DOI: 10.1681/ASN.2015080915

[81] Wang F, Lu X, Peng K, Fang H, Zhou L, Su J, et al. Antidiuretic action of collecting duct (pro)renin receptor downstream of vasopressin and PGE2 receptor EP4. Journal of the American Society of Nephrology. 2016;**27**(10):3022-3034. DOI: 10.1681/ASN.2015050592

[82] Nielsen S, Frøkiaer J, Marples D, Kwon TH, Agre P, Knepper MA. Aquaporins in the kidney: From molecules to medicine. Physiological Reviews. 2002;**82**(1):205-244. DOI: 10.1152/physrev.00024.2001

[83] Wynn TA. Cellular and molecular mechanisms of fibrosis. The Journal of Pathology. 2008;**214**(2):199-210. DOI: 10.1002/path.2277

[84] Wynn TA, Ramalingam TR. Mechanisms of fibrosis: Therapeutic translation for fibrotic disease. Nature Medicine. 2012;**18**(7):1028-1040. DOI: 10.1038/nm.2807

[85] He M, Zhang L, Shao Y, Wang X, Huang Y, Yao T, et al. Inhibition of renin/ prorenin receptor attenuated mesangial cell proliferation and reduced associated fibrotic factor release. European Journal of Pharmacology. 2009;**606**(1-3):155-161. DOI: 10.1016/j.ejphar.2008.12.050

[86] Ichihara A, Kaneshiro Y, Takemitsu T, Sakoda M, Suzuki F, Nakagawa T, et al. Nonproteolytic activation of prorenin contributes to development of cardiac fibrosis in genetic hypertension. Hypertension. 2006;**47**(5):894-900. DOI: 10.1161/01. HYP.0000215838.48170.0b

[87] Ishii K, Takeuchi H, Fukunaga K, Hirano Y, Suda K, Hagiwara T, et al. Attenuation of lipopolysaccharide-induced acute lung injury after (pro) renin receptor blockade. Experimental Lung Research. 2015;**41**(4):199-207. DOI: 10.3109/01902148.2014.993444

[88] Dong Y, Kanda A, Noda K, Saito W, Ishida S. Pathologic roles of receptor-associated prorenin system in idiopathic epiretinal membrane. Scientific Reports. 2017;7:44266. DOI: 10.1038/srep44266

[89] Li Z, Zhou L, Wang Y, Miao J, Hong X, Hou FF, et al. (Pro)renin receptor is an amplifier of Wnt/β-catenin signaling in kidney injury and fibrosis. Journal of the American Society of Nephrology. 2017;**28**(8):2393-2408. DOI: 10.1681/ASN.2016070811

[90] Liu Y, Zuo S, Li X, Fan J, Cao X, Yu X, et al. Interaction between V-ATPase B2 and (pro) renin receptors in promoting the progression of renal tubulointerstitial fibrosis. Scientific

Reports. 2016;**6**:25035. DOI: 10.1038/srep25035. Erratum in: Sci Rep. 2016;6:27677. doi: 10.1038/srep27677

[91] Jessup M, Brozena S. Heart failure. The New England Journal of Medicine. 2003;**348**:2007-2018. DOI: 10.1056/NEJMra021498

[92] Jiang F, Yang J, Zhang Y, Dong M, Wang S, Zhang Q, et al. Angiotensin-converting enzyme 2 and angiotensin 1-7: Novel therapeutic targets. Nature Reviews. Cardiology. 2014;**11**:413-426. DOI: 10.1038/nrcardio.2014.59

[93] Ellmers LJ, Rademaker MT, Charles CJ, Yandle TG, Richards AM. (Pro)renin receptor blockade ameliorates cardiac injury and remodeling and improves function after myocardial infarction. Journal of Cardiac Failure. 2016;**22**:64-72. DOI: 10.1016/j.cardfail.2015.08.341

[94] Yoshida A, Kanamori H, Naruse G, Minatoguchi S, Iwasa M, Yamada Y, et al. (Pro)renin receptor blockade ameliorates heart failure caused by chronic kidney disease. Journal of Cardiac Failure. 2019;**25**(4):286-300. DOI: 10.1016/j.cardfail.2019.02.009

[95] Zhang J, Cheng YJ, Luo CJ, Yu J. Inhibitory effect of (PRO)renin receptor decoy inhibitor PRO20 on endoplasmic reticulum stress during cardiac remodeling. Frontiers in Pharmacology. 2022;**13**:940365. DOI: 10.3389/fphar.2022.940365

[96] Li L, Cui YJ, Liu Y, Li HX, Su YD, Li SN, et al. ATP6AP2 knockdown in cardiomyocyte deteriorates heart function via compromising autophagic flux and NLRP3 inflammasome activation. Cell Death Discovery. 2022;**8**(1):161. DOI: 10.1038/s41420-022-00967-w

[97] Liu Y, Zhang S, Su D, Liu J, Cheng Y, Zou L, et al. Inhibiting (pro)renin receptor-mediated p38 MAPK signaling decreases hypoxia/reoxygenation-induced apoptosis in H9c2 cells. Molecular and Cellular Biochemistry. 2015;**403**(1-2):267-276. DOI: 10.1007/s11010-015-2356-8

[98] Gao X, Zhang S, Wang D, Cheng Y, Jiang Y, Liu Y. (Pro)renin receptor contributes to hypoxia/reoxygenation-induced apoptosis and autophagy in myocardial cells via the beta-catenin signaling pathway. Physiological Research. 2020;**69**(3):427-438. DOI: 10.33549/physiolres.934210

[99] Björkegren JLM, Lusis AJ. Atherosclerosis: Recent developments. Cell. 2022;**185**(10):1630-1645. DOI: 10.1016/j.cell.2022.04.004

[100] Mundi S, Massaro M, Scoditti E, Carluccio MA, van Hinsbergh VWM, Iruela-Arispe ML, et al. Endothelial permeability, LDL deposition, and cardiovascular risk factors-a review. Cardiovascular Research. 2018;**114**(1):35-52. DOI: 10.1093/cvr/cvx226

[101] Holmes MV, Asselbergs FW, Palmer TM, Drenos F, Lanktree MB, Nelson CP, et al. Mendelian randomization of blood lipids for coronary heart disease. European Heart Journal. 2015;**36**(9):539-550. DOI: 10.1093/eurheartj/eht571

[102] Lu X, Meima ME, Nelson JK, Sorrentino V, Loregger A, Scheij S, et al. Identification of the (pro)renin receptor as a novel regulator of low-density lipoprotein metabolism. Circulation Research. 2016;**118**(2):222-229. DOI: 10.1161/CIRCRESAHA.115.306799

[103] Strong A, Musunuru K. (Pro)renin receptor and LDL clearance: An old player joins a new game. Circulation

Research. 2016;**118**(2):187-189. DOI: 10.1161/CIRCRESAHA.115.308068

[104] Ren L, Sun Y, Lu H, Ye D, Han L, Wang N, et al. (Pro)renin receptor inhibition reprograms hepatic lipid metabolism and protects mice from diet-induced obesity and hepatosteatosis. Circulation Research. 2018;**122**(5):730-741. DOI: 10.1161/CIRCRESAHA.117.312422

[105] Batenburg WW, Krop M, Garrelds IM, de Vries R, de Bruin RJ, Burcklé CA, et al. Prorenin is the endogenous agonist of the (pro)renin receptor. Binding kinetics of renin and prorenin in rat vascular smooth muscle cells overexpressing the human (pro) renin receptor. Journal of Hypertension. 2007;**25**(12):2441-2453. DOI: 10.1097/HJH.0b013e3282f05bae

[106] Greco CM, Camera M, Facchinetti L, Brambilla M, Pellegrino S, Gelmi ML, et al. Chemotactic effect of prorenin on human aortic smooth muscle cells: A novel function of the (pro) renin receptor. Cardiovascular Research. 2012;**95**(3):366-374. DOI: 10.1093/cvr/cvs204

[107] Ma H, Dong XF, Cao XR, Hei NH, Li JL, Wang YL, et al. Pro-renin receptor overexpression promotes angiotensin II-induced abdominal aortic aneurysm formation in apolipoprotein E-knockout mice. Human Gene Therapy. 2020;**31**(11-12):639-650. DOI: 10.1089/hum.2019.124

[108] Li C, Siragy HM. High glucose induces podocyte injury via enhanced (pro)renin receptor-Wnt-β-catenin-snail signaling pathway. PLoS One. 2014;**9**(2):e89233. DOI: 10.1371/journal.pone.0089233

[109] Oshima Y, Morimoto S, Ichihara A. Roles of the (pro)renin receptor in the kidney. World Journal of Nephrology. 2014;**3**(4):302-307. DOI: 10.5527/wjn.v3.i4.302

[110] Ishizawa K, Yoshizumi M, Tsuchiya K, Takishita E, Nakaya Y, Kishi K, et al. Effects of losartan in combination with or without exercise on insulin resistance in Otsuka long-Evans Tokushima fatty rats. European Journal of Pharmacology. 2001;**430**:359-367. DOI: 10.1016/S0014-2999(01)01405-4

[111] Samad F, Yamamoto K, Pandey M, Loskutoff DJ. Elevated expression of transforming growth factor-beta in adipose tissue from obese mice. Molecular Medicine. 1997;**3**:37-48. [PMID: 9132278]

[112] Balakrishnan S, Sadasivam M, Kannan A, Panneerselvam A, Prahalathan C. Glucose modulates Pax6 expression through the JNK/p38 MAP kinase pathway in pancreatic betacells. Life Sciences. 2014;**109**:1-7. DOI: 10.1016/j.lfs.2014.06.009

[113] Youl E, Magous R, Cros G, Oiry C. MAP kinase cross talks involvement in the protective activity of quercetin. Fundamental & Clinical Pharmacology. 2014;**28**:608-615. DOI: 10.1111/fcp.12078

[114] El Khattabi I, Sharma A. Preventing p38 MAPK-mediated MafA degradation ameliorates β-cell dysfunction under oxidative stress. Molecular Endocrinology. 2013;**27**:1078-1090. DOI: 10.1210/me.2012-1346

[115] Bokuda K, Ichihara A. Possible contribution of (pro)renin receptor to development of gestational diabetes mellitus. World Journal of Diabetes. 2014;**5**(6):912-916. DOI: 10.4239/wjd.v5.i6.912

[116] Sun-Wada GH, Toyomura T, Murata Y, Yamamoto A, Futai M, Wada Y. The a3 isoform of V-ATPase

regulates insulin secretion from pancreatic beta-cells. Journal of Cell Science. 2006;**119**:4531-4540. DOI: 10.1242/jcs.03234

[117] Choi YO, Park JH, Song YS, Lee W, Moriyama Y, Choe H, et al. Involvement of vesicular H+-ATPase in insulin-stimulated glucose transport in 3T3-F442A adipocytes. Endocrine Journal. 2007;**54**:733-743. DOI: 10.1507/endocrj.K07-090

[118] Huang J, Ledford KJ, Pitkin WB, Russo L, Najjar SM, Siragy HM. Targeted deletion of murine CEACAM 1 activates PI3K-Akt signaling and contributes to the expression of (pro)renin receptor via CREB family and NF-kappaB transcription factors. Hypertension. 2013;**62**(2):317-323. DOI: 10.1161/HYPERTENSIONAHA.113.01324

[119] Wang J, Shibayama Y, Zhang A, Ohsaki H, Asano E, Suzuki Y, et al. (Pro) renin receptor promotes colorectal cancer through the Wnt/beta-catenin signalling pathway despite constitutive pathway component mutations. British Journal of Cancer. 2019;**120**(2):229-237. DOI: 10.1038/s41416-018-0350-0

[120] Arundhathi A, Chuang WH, Chen JK, Wang SE, Shyr YM, Chen JY, et al. Prorenin receptor acts as a potential molecular target for pancreatic ductal adenocarcinoma diagnosis. Oncotarget. 2016;**7**(34):55437-55448. DOI: 10.18632/oncotarget.10583

[121] Kouchi M, Shibayama Y, Ogawa D, Miyake K, Nishiyama A, Tamiya T. (Pro)renin receptor is crucial for glioma development via the Wnt/beta-catenin signaling pathway. Journal of Neurosurgery. 2017;**127**:819-828. DOI: 10.3171/2016.9.JNS16431

[122] Ohba K, Suzuki T, Nishiyama H, Kaneko K, Hirose T, Totsune K, et al. Expression of (pro)renin receptor in breast cancers and its effect on cancer cell proliferation. Biomedical Research. 2014;**35**:117-126. DOI: 10.2220/biomedres.35.117

[123] Yamamoto H, Kaneko K, Ohba K, Morimoto R, Hirose T, Satoh F, et al. Increased expression of (pro) renin receptor in aldosterone-producing adenomas. Peptides. 2013;**49**:68-73. DOI: 10.1016/j.peptides.2013.08.022

[124] Shibayama Y, Fujimori T, Nguyen G, Hirose T, Totsune K, Ichihara A, et al. (Pro)renin receptor is crucial for Wnt/beta-catenin-dependent genesis of pancreatic ductal adenocarcinoma. Scientific Reports. 2015;**5**:8854. DOI: 10.1038/srep08854

[125] Delforce SJ, Lumbers ER, Corbisier de Meaultsart C, Wang Y, Proietto A, Otton G, et al. Expression of renin-angiotensin system (RAS) components in endometrial cancer. Endocrine Connections. 2017;**6**(1):9-19. DOI: 10.1530/EC-16-0082

[126] Juillerat-Jeanneret L, Celerier J, Chapuis Bernasconi C, Nguyen G, Wostl W, Maerki HP, et al. Renin and angiotensinogen expression and functions in growth and apoptosis of human glioblastoma. British Journal of Cancer. 2004;**90**(5):1059-1068. DOI: 10.1038/sj.bjc.6601646

[127] Morimoto S, Ando T, Niiyama M, Seki Y, Yoshida N, Watanabe D, et al. Serum soluble (pro)renin receptor levels in patients with essential hypertension. Hypertension Research. 2014;**37**:642-648. DOI: 10.1038/hr.2014.46

[128] Wang F, Xu C, Luo R, Peng K, Ramkumar N, Xie S, et al. Site-1 protease-derived soluble (pro)renin receptor targets vasopressin receptor 2 to enhance urine concentrating

capability. JCI Insight. 2019;**4**(7):e124174. DOI: 10.1172/jci.insight.124174

[129] Ramkumar N, Stuart D, Peterson CS, Hu C, Wheatley W, Min Cho J, et al. Loss of soluble (pro)renin receptor attenuates angiotensin-ii induced hypertension and renal injury. Circulation Research. 2021;**129**:50-62. DOI: 10.1161/CIRCRESAHA.120.317532

[130] Fu Z, Wang F, Liu X, Hu J, Su J, Lu X, et al. Soluble (pro)renin receptor induces endothelial dysfunction and hypertension in mice with diet-induced obesity via activation of angiotensin II type 1 receptor. Clinical Science. 2021;**135**(6):793-810. DOI: 10.1042/CS20201047

[131] Obradovic D, Loncar G, Radenovic S, Tahirovic E, Heidecke H, Schulze-Forster K, et al. Soluble (pro) renin receptor in elderly chronic heart failure patients. Frontiers in Bioscience. 2020;**25**(10):1839-1853. DOI: 10.2741/4880

[132] Xue K, Wang Y, Wang Y, Fang H. Advanced oxidation protein product promotes oxidative accentuation in renal epithelial cells via the soluble (pro) renin receptor-mediated intrarenal renin-angiotensin system and Nox4-H_2O_2 signaling. Oxidative Medicine and Cellular Longevity. 2021;**2021**:5710440. DOI: 10.1155/2021/5710440

[133] Gong L, Zhang S, Li L, Gao X, Wang D, Wu D, et al. Elevated plasma soluble (pro)renin receptor levels are associated with left ventricular remodeling and renal function in chronic heart failure patients with reduced ejection fraction. Peptides. 2019;**111**:152-157. DOI: 10.1016/j.peptides.2018.04.010

[134] Lumbers ER, Pringle KG. Roles of the circulating renin-angiotensin-aldosterone system in human pregnancy. American Journal of Physiology. Regulatory, Integrative and Comparative Physiology. 2014;**306**:R91-R101. DOI: 10.1152/ajpregu.00034.2013

[135] Chesley LC. Hypertensive Disorders in Pregnancy. Appleton-Century Crofts. Center for Biology and Society - Arizona State University; 1978

[136] Seldin D, Giebisch G. Kidney Physiology and Pathology. New York: Raven Press; 1992. p. 3

[137] Duley L. The global impact of pre-eclampsia and eclampsia. Seminars in Perinatology. 2009;**33**(3):130-137. DOI: 10.1053/j.semperi.2009.02.010. PMID: 19464502

[138] Schofield LG, Endacott SK, Delforce SJ, Lumbers ER, Pringle KG. Importance of the (pro)renin receptor in activating the renin-angiotensin system during normotensive and preeclamptic pregnancies. Current Hypertension Reports. 2024;**26**:483-495. DOI: 10.1007/s11906-024-01316-1

[139] Watanabe N, Bokuda K, Fujiwar T, Suzuki T, Mito A, Morimoto S, et al. Soluble (pro)renin receptor and blood pressure during pregnancy: A prospective cohort study. Hypertension. 2012;**60**:1250-1256. DOI: 10.1161/HYPERTENSIONAHA.112.197418

[140] Narita T, Ichihara A, Matsuoka K, Takai Y, Bokuda K, Morimoto S, et al. Placental (pro) renin receptor expression and plasma soluble (pro) renin receptor levels in preeclampsia. Placenta. 2016;**37**:72-78. DOI: 10.1016/j.placenta.2015.11.007

[141] Mistry H, Kurlak L, Pipkin FB. The placental renin–angiotensin system and oxidative stress in pre-eclampsia. Placenta. 2013;**34**:182-186. DOI: 10.1016/j.placenta.2012.11.027

[142] Shah DM, Banu JM, Chirgwin JM, Tekmal RR. Reproductive tissue renin gene expression in preeclampsia. Hypertension in Pregnancy. 2000;**19**:341-351. DOI: 10.1081/prg-100101996

[143] Schofield LG, Delforce SJ, Pryor JC, Endacott SK, Lumbers ER, Marshall SA, et al. The soluble (pro) renin receptor promotes a preeclampsia-like phenotype both *in vitro* and *in vivo*. Hypertension Research. 2024:**47**(6):1627-1641. DOI: 10.1038/s41440-024-01678-8

[144] Verdonk K, Visser W, Van Den Meiracker AH, Danser AH. The renin-angiotensin-aldosterone system in pre-eclampsia: The delicate balance between good and bad. Clinical Science (London, England). 2014;**126**(8):537-544. DOI: 10.1042/CS20130455

[145] Zhou A, Carrell RW, Murphy MP, Wei Z, Yan Y, Stanley PL, et al. A redox switch in angiotensinogen modulates angiotensin release. Nature. 2010;**468**(7320):108-111. DOI: 10.1038/nature09505

[146] Quitterer U, Lother H, Abdalla S. AT1 receptor heterodimers and angiotensin II responsiveness in preeclampsia. Seminars in Nephrology. 2004;**24**(2):115-119. DOI: 10.1016/j.semnephrol.2003.11.007

[147] Xia Y, Kellems RE. Angiotensin receptor agonistic autoantibodies and hypertension: Preeclampsia and beyond. Circulation Research. 2013;**113**:78-87. DOI: 10.1161/CIRCRESAHA.113.300752

[148] Zou LX, Imig JD, von Thun AM, Hymel A, Ono H, Navar LG. Receptor-mediated intrarenal angiotensin II augmentation in angiotensin II–infused rats. Hypertension. 1996;**28**:669-677. DOI: 10.1161/01.hyp.28.4.669

[149] Nishiyama A, Seth DM, Navar LG. Renal interstitial fluid concentrations of angiotensins I and II in anesthetized rats. Hypertension. 2002;**39**:129-134. DOI: 10.1161/hy0102.100536

[150] Wang Y, Wang Y, Xue K, Wang H, Zhou J, Gao F, et al. (Pro) renin receptor antagonist PRO20 attenuates nephrectomy-induced nephropathy in rats via inhibition of intrarenal RAS and Wnt/β-catenin signaling. Physiological Reports. 2021;**9**(11):e14881. DOI: 10.14814/phy2.14881

[151] Wang J, Nishiyama A, Matsuyama M, Wang Z, Yuan Y. The (pro)renin receptor: A novel biomarker and potential therapeutic target for various cancers. Cell Communication and Signaling: CCS. 2020;**18**:39. DOI: 10.1186/s12964-020-0531-3

[152] Maruyama N, Segawa T, Kinoshita N, Ichihara A. Novel sandwich ELISA for detecting the human soluble (pro) renin receptor. Frontiers in Bioscience (Elite Edition). 2013;**5**:583-590. DOI: 10.2741/e640

[153] Fukushima A, Kinugawa S, Homma T, Masaki Y, Furihata T, Abe T, et al. Increased plasma soluble (pro) renin receptor levels are correlated with renal dysfunction in patients with heart failure. International Journal of Cardiology. 2013;**168**:4313-4314. DOI: 10.1016/j.ijcard.2013.04.176

[154] Hamada K, Taniguchi Y, Shimamura Y, Inoue K, Ogata K, Ishihara M, et al. Serum level of soluble (pro) renin receptor is modulated in chronic kidney disease. Clinical and Experimental Nephrology. 2013;**17**:848-856. DOI: 10.1007/s10157-013-0803-y

[155] Kaneshiro Y, Ichihara A, Sakoda M, Takemitsu TY, Nabi AN, Uddin M, et al. Slowly progressive, angiotensin

II-independent glomerulosclerosis in human (pro)renin receptor-transgenic rats. Journal of the American Society of Nephrology: JASN. 2007;**18**(6):1789-1795. DOI: 10.1681/ASN.2006091062

[156] Larrinaga G, Calvete-Candenas J, Solano-Iturri JD, Martín AM, Pueyo A, Nunes-Xavier CE, et al. (Pro)renin receptor is a novel independent prognostic marker in invasive urothelial carcinoma of the bladder. Cancers. 2021;**13**(22):5642. DOI: 10.3390/cancers13225642

[157] Beitia M, Solano-Iturri JD, Errarte P, Calvete-Candenas J, Loizate A, Etxezarraga MC, et al. (pro) renin receptor expression increases throughout the colorectal adenoma-adenocarcinoma sequence and it is associated with worse colorectal cancer prognosis. Cancers (Basel). 2019;**11**(6):881. DOI: 10.3390/cancers11060881

[158] Kreienbring K, Franz A, Richter R, Dragun D, Heidecke H, Dechend R, et al. Predictive and prognostic value of sPRR in patients with primary epithelial ovarian cancer. Analytical Cellular Pathology (Amsterdam). 2016;**2016**:6845213. DOI: 10.1155/2016/6845213

Chapter 4

Angiotensin-Converting Enzyme and Blood Basic Carboxypeptidases CPB2 and CPN Activity is an Indicator for Serum Quality: A Quick Lab Test

Vivien Osterhus and Simone König

Abstract

The vasoactive neuropeptide bradykinin (BK) is involved in major pathophysiological pathways such as the kinin-kallikrein system (KKS) and the renin-angiotensin system (RAS). It is a substrate of important enzymes, namely angiotensin-converting enzyme (ACE) and basic carboxypeptidases N (CPN) and B2 (CPB2). We use its dabsylated form (DBK) as a reporter substance to monitor the serum activity of these proteases. The activity of the enzymes is responsible for the formation of two DBK fragments, which can be detected with this neuropeptide reporter assay (NRA) to elucidate disease-related changes in RAS and KKS. The assay is also sensitive to serum quality. Hemolytic serum shows significantly reduced serum protease activity in the NRA, but it can already be visually identified by its colour. With the NRA, we detected samples from healthy controls, which were not visibly hemolytic and still exhibited the same poor results. This observation was traced back to lax use of the sampling protocol in the clinic. The incorporation of such samples of poor serum quality in biochemical studies would impact on their outcome and reproducibility. Thus, we have simplified the NRA workflow in order to generate a quick test, which can help to weed out samples of poor quality.

Keywords: neuropeptide reporter assay, dabsylated bradykinin, serum protease activity, ACE, COVID-19

1. Introduction

1.1 Bradykinin as reporter substance

The neuropeptide bradykinin (BK, sequence RPPGFSPFR) is important in blood pressure homeostasis and it is associated with the inflammatory response and vascular permeability functions including thrombosis and blood coagulation [1]. BK is a substrate of angiotensin-converting enzyme (ACE) [2] and basic carboxypeptidases

N (CPN) [3] and B2 (CPB2, also known as thrombin activatable fibrinolysis inhibitor (TAFI), CPU and pCPB [4–7]). These enzymes are interconnected in the major physiological pathways kinin-kallikrein system (KKS), renin-angiotensin system (RAS) and fibrinolysis (**Figure 1**) [2, 3, 8].

In the KKS, vasoactive BK is formed from kininogen by the action of kallikrein. ACE deactivates BK and cleaves angiotensin (Ang) I to Ang II. In the classical RAS, Ang II binds to its receptors type 1 and 2 (AT1R, AT2R) with opposite effects on, among other functions, blood pressure and inflammation. The main antagonist to the classical RAS is ACE2, which removes Ang II by cleavage to Ang(1-7); this peptide binds to the Mas receptor, thereby reducing blood pressure [2]. ACE2 became also of interest as severe acute respiratory syndrome coronavirus 2 (SARS-CoV-2) receptor in the recent COVID-19 pandemic [8, 14, 15].

BK acts via receptors B1 and B2. Cleavage of BK by carboxypeptidases changes receptor specificity from B2R to B1R [9–12]. CPN and CPB2 degrade BK to des-Arg9-BK [3, 12], which is deactivated by ACE2. CPB2 reduces fibrinolysis by fibrin

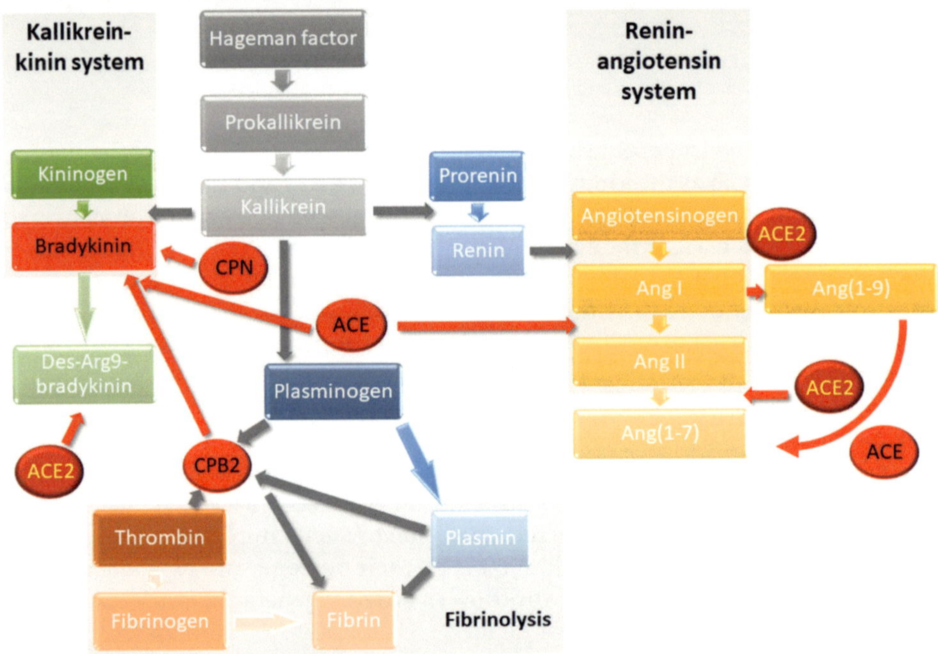

Figure 1.
Interplay of the KKS, RAS and fibrinolysis with regard to BK, the reporter peptide in the NRA [2, 3, 8]. Vasoactive BK is formed from kininogen by the action of kallikrein. The latter needs the Hageman factor to be cleaved from its precursor, and it also influences the RAS by catalyzing the cleavage of prorenin to renin, which, in turn, assists the formation of Ang I from angiotensinogen. The generation of Ang II ensures blood pressure homeostasis and is counter-balanced by ACE2, which cleaves Ang II and acts also as a SARS-CoV2 receptor. KKS and RAS are further connected by the action of ACE, which deactivates BK and cleaves Ang I to Ang II. In the classical RAS, Ang II binds to its receptors AT1R and AT2R with opposite effects on, among other functions, blood pressure and inflammation. The main antagonist to the classical RAS is ACE2, which removes Ang II by cleavage to Ang (1–7); this peptide binds to the Mas receptor, thereby reducing blood pressure. BK acts via receptors B1 and B2. Cleavage of BK by carboxypeptidases changes receptor specificity from B2R to B1R [9–12]. CPN and CPB2 degrade BK to des-Arg9-BK, which is deactivated by ACE2. CPB2 circulates in the plasma as plasminogen-bound zymogen and is activated by proteolysis by the thrombin/thrombomodulin complex. CPB2 reduces fibrinolysis by removing the fibrin C-terminal residues that are important for the binding and activation of plasminogen [4, 12]. Plasmin is generated from plasminogen; it is present in blood and degrades many proteins including fibrin clots (fibrinolysis) [13]. Molecules of interest for the NRA (BK, ACE, CPN, CPB2) are colored in red.

cleavage [4, 12]. Looking at these complex relationships, it is not surprising that this enzyme network is a research target in many cardiovascular and inflammatory diseases [10, 11, 16].

1.2 Neuropeptide reporter assay

We have been interested in BK in the context of pain and have used its dabsylated form (DBK) as a reporter substance to monitor patient serum protease activity in Complex-Regional Pain Syndrome (CRPS) [17–19]. The dabsyl-label at the N-terminus of the peptide introduces an orange color to the molecule so that all cleavage fragments carrying the label are visible to the naked eye. They can be separated by the low-tech robust analytical technique thin-layer chromatography (TLC) and be used to study enzyme activity.

In our neuropeptide reporter assay (NRA) [17], we incubate DBK with serum and separate the generated peptide fragments by TLC (for workflow and exemplary results, see **Figure 2**). Thereby, ACE cleaves DBK (also called DBK1-9 for indication of the peptide length) at position 5–6, leading to the formation of fragment DBK1-5, while CPN and CPB2 are responsible for the generation of fragment DBK1-8. Using this tool, we have shown that the ACE serum activity was compromised in patients with CRPS, a disease where symptoms develop locally [18].

We have also studied hospitalized and convalescent COVID-19 patients and found that DBK cleavage was generally impaired in hospitalized patients. Carboxypeptidase activity was significantly reduced [20–22]. The DBK cleavage product generated by ACE, fragment 1–5 (DBK1-5), was increased in critically ill patients and strongly correlated with clinical heart and liver parameters. Experimental values returned to normal levels during convalescence in the majority of patients, but a number of probands showed similar results as measured in hospitalized patients so that we hypothesized

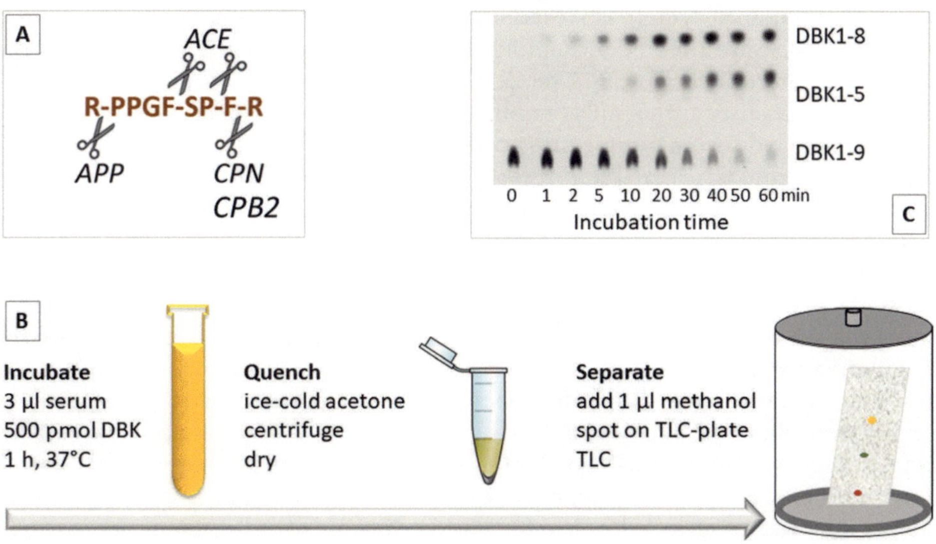

Figure 2.
(A) Structure of BK and enzyme cleavage sites. (B) Workflow of the NRA using DBK (DBK1–9, for details on incubation and TLC separation, see [17]). (C) Exemplary TLC plate showing a 1 hour time course for DBK degradation by serum of a healthy control.

that dysregulated CPN/CPB2 and ACE serum activity could be an indication for the development of Long COVID [22].

Currently, we are using the NRA in a study of the RAS in inflammatory skin diseases. The assay is a great tool in any investigation that targets enzymes such as ACE and CPN specifically, or complex systems like RAS and KKS generally. It is valuable in clinical research, but not yet implemented in diagnostics.

In addition, we found the NRA useful for a completely different purpose, namely an activity test for snake venom proteases when studying the inhibitory properties of plant material [23]. Venom metalloproteinases degraded DBK in a few minutes.

1.3 Serum quality control

Serum is normally clear and straw colored [24]. Occasionally, we are supplied with orange-red or turbid-opaque (or a combination of both) sera. The lysis of red blood cells is responsible for the coloring, while lipemia causes the milky white appearance. The most common cause of lipemia is food intake shortly before the blood draw, but there are also medical conditions such as hypertriglyceridemia causing the effect [24]. Hemolysis is mostly (50–70% of cases [24]) associated with the phlebotomy technique and the skill of the medical personnel (use of narrow gauge needles, forceful use of syringe, overly vigorous shaking of blood tube, delays in processing, etc. [24, 25]), but there are rare cases of in vivo hemolysis to be considered (2% [26]).

We observed in different projects that the NRA was sensitive to serum quality. It was not surprising that hemolytic sera did not exhibit the same protease activity in the NRA compared to serum of good quality; DBK was hardly cleaved and the intensity of the DBK fragments was significantly lower than expected. Clearly, erythrocyte lysis and the release of the cell content including proteases into the blood changes the serum composition drastically and impacts on laboratory testing and biochemical measurements such as our enzyme activity experiments. This phenomenon is a major challenge when selecting or rejecting samples for testing [24, 26]. It is well documented that standard protein lab tests such as lactate dehydrogenase and aspartate aminotransferase are affected by hemolysis, but even minerals like potassium cannot be correctly determined [26–32]. The Centers for Disease Control and Prevention (CDC) [33] and other authors [34] published hemolysis charts according to which deep orange to red serum samples are not fit for analysis. Visual inspection is however subjective [35] and larger labs thus ressort to spectrophotometric analysis for evaluation of the degree of hemolysis [24, 36–38] or even deep learning [39].

Interestingly and even more importantly, using the NRA, we also noted lower protease activity in some visually non-hemolytic sera obtained from our clinic for the COVID-19 study [21]. Measurements for healthy controls did not agree with earlier results and were, in fact, way off, similar to hemolytic samples. On our insistence that something must have gone wrong during sampling, the results were eventually traced back to the random use of different collection tubes by the medical staff and new samples were obtained. This was not a single event; a batch of low-performing non-hemolytic serum samples was also identified from one group in a large multi-center study (unpublished). In that case, it was even more surprising, because all involved collaborators were aware of the need for standardization of collection procedures. The reason for the discrepancy remains unknown. We found it subsequently very helpful to use our NRA as a tool to evaluate the quality of the sera given to us. It is a quick and low-cost method to avoid the inclusion of samples of poor quality as a result of human error in more expensive studies such as omics experiments [40, 41]. Data obtained from such samples would influence the study outcome by generating unreproducible results. In contrast to hemolytic samples, the NRA was not sensitive to lipemic serum; the results for DBK cleavage fell into the expected ranges.

1.4 Aim

The above-mentioned clinical studies have shown the usefulness of our protease activity test using DBK degradation as a signal in biochemical research. Soon, the idea was born to simplify the NRA workflow and design an easy, robust, and quick assay for wide applicability. It was nurtured by the observation that the NRA can weed out poor quality, non-hemolytic serum samples from study cohorts. For quality control, it is even more important to have a fast and simple way of testing. Therefore, we evaluated, if we can simplify the NRA workflow using as little as possible of any laboratory equipment.

2. Experimental

Blood was obtained from healthy volunteers observing the declaration of Helsinki. Ethical permission for the study [18] was granted from the IRB of the Rhineland–Palatinate Medical Association (registration number 4208). The standard NRA workflow has been described in Ref. [17] (**Figure 2**). Briefly, 3 µl serum was incubated with dried DBK at 37°C for a desired time period, typically 1 hour. The process was stopped by adding ice-cold acetone and freezing for min—3 hours. Then, the solution was centrifuged and the supernatant dried. For TLC, the supernatant was resuspended in methanol. TLC silica gel 60 sheets (20 x 20 cm) as used in Ref. [17] were purchased from Merck Millipore (Darmstadt, Germany) and so were the TLC aluminum sheets with concentration zone (silica gel 60, 20 x 2.5 cm). This protocol was simplified as described below.

3. Results and discussion

The NRA has been extensively validated in the original publication [17]. Here, several steps in the NRA protocol were evaluated to simplify the workflow including incubation time and temperature, quenching and TLC. We could show that a 15 minutes incubation of serum with DBK at 37°C was sufficient to obtain visual evidence of the degradation of DBK1-9 and the formation of DBK1-8, which was needed to use the assay for quality control purposes. Serum of low quality will hardly cleave DBK1-9, and this evidence can be obtained in a short period of time. Fragment DBK1-5 tends to be less abundant and can be better visualized by scanning [17]. At room temperature (RT), the enzyme activity was not much compromised, but to be safe, the incubation time was extended to 30 minutes. Subsequently, the sample was diluted with 3 µl methanol, vortexed (VortexGenie 2, Scientific Instruments), and briefly centrifuged using a small bench device (Sprout, Biozyme), a process, which hardly took 3 minutes.

Instead of a regular TLC chamber, we used a 50 ml Falcon tube for sample separation. The elution solvent (chloroform, 1.1 ml; methanol, 400 µl; water, 60 µl; formic acid, 9 µl, as described [17]) was placed in the cap of the Falcon tube. The tube was screwed to its top and left standing upright for 30 minutes for saturation of the chamber; this step could optionally be eliminated. The commercial TLC plate was cut to a size of 2 x 10 cm and the sample was spotted at ~1.5 cm from the edge of the plate. The spot was left to dry on the bench for ~5 minutes, and then the plate was placed in the Falcon tube (**Figure 3C**). TLC proceeded at RT and was stopped when the solvent front almost reached the upper edge of the plate (~1 cm distance). The plate was briefly dried using a common hairdryer. Typical results are shown in **Figure 3A,B** and they are reproducible. TLC spots were enlarged and not as well defined as in the optimized protocol, but of sufficient quality to allow grading.

The experiments demonstrated that it is possible to cut a few corners in the assay in order to simplify the protocol for quick testing (**Table 1**). Specifically, the incubation time could be reduced by half or even more, depending, on if the incubation proceeded at RT or if the temperature was controlled. While analyte separation was

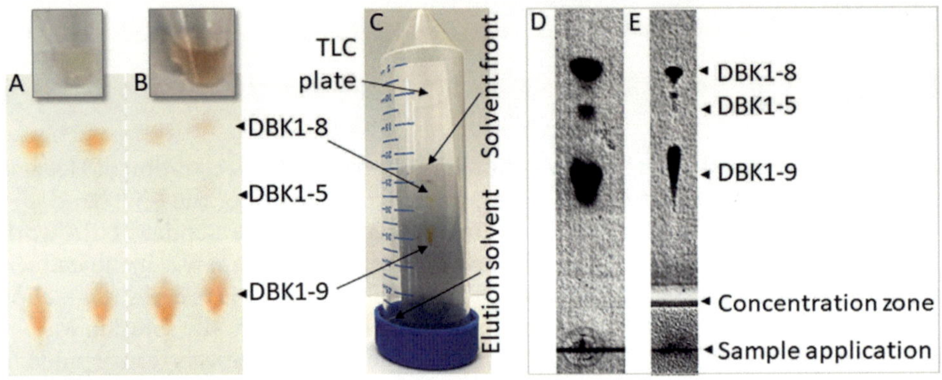

Figure 3.
Results (A/B) and set-up (C) of the simplified NRA workflow (37°C, 15 minutes incubation) for a normal (A) and a hemolytic (B) serum, which can be recognized by its red color. A/B) Photographs of TLC plates showing the intact DBK and the major fragment DBK1-8. DBK1-8 spots from hemolytic serum (B) exhibit less intensity than those from normal serum (A); vice versa for DBK1-9. Fragment DBK1-5 is better seen in a scan of the TLC plate (D/E). (C) A Falcon tube is used instead of a regular TLC chamber. Commercial TLC plates are manually cut to fit. (D/E) Scans of TLC plates to illustrate the difference in spot size obtained with a regular TLC plate (D) and a TLC plate with a concentration zone (E).

Protocol step	Validated NRA [17]	Time	Quick test	Time
Incubation	37°C	1 h	37°C (or RT, 30 minutes)	15 minutes
Extraction	Protein precipitation with acetone, freeze, centrifuge, dry, redissolve in 3 µl	> 3 h	Addition of methanol, vortex, centrifuge (or SPE, ~ 5 minutes)	< 1 minutes
Application to TLC plate	3 x 1 µl	~ 2 min	1 x 6 µl	< 1 minutes
TLC plates	Regular		With concentration zone	
TLC	Commercial chamber		Falcon tube	
Spot size	Well controlled		Slightly enlarged	
Results	Quantitative		Semi-quantitative	

Table 1.
Comparison of protocol steps of the validated NRA and the simplified workflow. The quick test generates results in a fraction of the time necessary for the validated workflow [17] and allows to semi-quantitatively evaluate the quality of the sample.

not possible when directly applying the incubation mixture (3 µl serum + DBK) to the TLC plate, TLC could be performed after adding 3 µl of methanol to the mixture. The organic solvent collected the labeled fragments and separated them from serum matrix components so that they became accessible for the chromatographic run. Protein precipitation with cold acetone was completely eliminated saving ~3 hours of freezing, centrifuging and drying. Clearly disadvantageous was the associated volume increase for sample application to the TLC plate. While before [17], we spotted the sample in three steps to the plate with intermittent drying of the spot on air to keep it small, we tested here, whether a single sample application was possible. Spot size and shape suffered, but not as much as expected. We also found TLC plates having a concentration zone useful in order to focus the spots more (**Figure 3D,E**).

Further, we have evaluated changes in other steps in the workflow, which might come in handy for specific applications. For instance, we used reversed-phase solid-phase extraction (SPE) on pipette tips (Zip-Tip C18 microbed, Millipore) to purify the analytes. To that end, 7 µl of an aqueous buffer was added to the incubation mixture before SPE. For elution from the SPE-tip, 5–10 µl of 75% methanol (with 25% water, and 1% formic acid) was used. This was another way of isolating the analytes from the serum background, but slightly more laborious.

We have shown before that the NRA can be performed both with whole blood and dried blood from blood cards [42]. This procedure can be simplified in a similar manner, but the blood needs to be diluted with buffer or water; otherwise, the DBK analytes cannot be properly separated from the blood components.

4. Conclusion

The measurement of the activity of proteases in serum or blood allows disease-dependent monitoring of selected physiological processes, in our case, KKS and RAS. For this purpose, we use labeled BK as a reporter molecule and detect the formation of its cleavage fragments by TLC. Earlier, we had developed and validated the NRA workflow [17], which we subsequently used in two clinical studies [18–22]. Interestingly, we also noted that the NRA was sensitive to serum quality, confidently picking out samples of low enzyme activity from healthy donors resulting, e.g., from thoughtless changes in sampling protocol. Thus, it can be used as a quality control assay when selecting or rejecting samples for larger and possibly expensive studies. Obviously, the test is only sensible with cohorts of healthy donors, because in patient cohorts, the DBK cleavage activity is expected to differ due to physiological processes.

We envisaged a NRA quick test both for research (outpatient) and quality control purposes. To that end, we simplified the workflow by reducing the lab time, protocol steps and the use of lab devices. This was possible with little information loss on the signals for the major analytes (DBK1-9, DBK1-8), but with limitations regarding the detection of the light signal for DBK1-5. Thus, we recommend to still use the optimized NRA protocol [22, 42, 43] for biochemical investigations and the shortened protocol for quick quality checks.

The ultimate goal was a completely independent-of-technical-devices NRA kit based on a procedure, which could be performed by laypersons. The work above was a major step in this direction, although we still rely on pipettes and bench centrifuges. TLC with analytes, which are visible to the naked eye, holds much promise for such endeavors due to its simple analytical principle.

Acknowledgements

The authors thank M. Bayer for collaboration on the NRA and F. Birklein for the joint work on CRPS. Publication was supported by the Open Access Fund of the University of Münster.

Conflict of interest

The authors declare no conflict of interest.

Abbreviations

ACE	angiotensin-converting enzyme
ACE2	angiotensin-converting enzyme 2
Ang	angiotensin
Ang(1-7)	angiotensin fragment 1-7
AT1R	angiotensin II receptor type 1
AT2R	angiotensin II receptor type 2
B1R	bradykinin receptor B1
B2R	bradykinin receptor B2
BK	bradykinin
COVID-19	coronavirus disease 2019
CPB2 (or TAFI, CPU, pCPB)	carboxypeptidase B2
CPN	carboxypeptidase N
CRPS	complex-regional pain syndrome
DBK (or DBK1-9)	dabsylated bradykinin
DBK1-5	dabsylated bradykinin fragment 1-5
DBK1-8	dabsylated bradykinin fragment 1-8
KKS	kinin-kallikrein system
NRA	neuropeptide reporter assay
RAS	renin-angiotensin system
RT	room temperature
SARS-CoV-2	severe acute respiratory syndrome coronavirus 2
SPE	solid-phase extraction
TLC	thin-layer chromatography

Author details

Vivien Osterhus and Simone König*
Core Unit Proteomics, Interdisciplinary Center for Clinical Research, University of Münster, Münster, Germany

*Address all correspondence to: koenigs@uni-muenster.de

References

[1] Rex DAB, Deepak K, Vaid N, Dagamajalu S, Kandasamy RK, Flo TH, et al. A modular map of bradykinin-mediated inflammatory signaling network. Journal of Cell Communication and Signaling. 2022;**16**:301-310. DOI: 10.1007/s12079-021-00652-0

[2] Paz Ocaranza M, Riquelme JA, García L, Jalil JE, Chiong M, Santos RAS, et al. Counter-regulatory renin-angiotensin system in cardiovascular disease. Nature Reviews. Cardiology. 2020;**17**:116-129. DOI: 10.1038/s41569-019-0244-8

[3] Matthews KW, Mueller-Ortiz SL, Wetsel RA. Carboxypeptidase N: A pleiotropic regulator of inflammation. Molecular Immunology. 2004;**40**:785-793. DOI: 10.1016/j.molimm.2003.10.002

[4] Sillen M, Declerck PJ. Thrombin activatable fibrinolysis inhibitor (TAFI): An updated narrative review. International Journal of Molecular Sciences. 2021;**22**:3670-3686. DOI: 10.3390/ijms22073670

[5] Claesen K, Mertens JC, Leenaerts D, Hendriks D. Carboxypeptidase U (CPU, TAFIa, CPB2) in thromboembolic disease: What do we know three decades after its discovery? International Journal of Molecular Sciences. 2021;**22**:883-914. DOI: 10.3390/ijms22020883

[6] Myles T, Nishimura T, Yun TH, Nagashima M, Morser J, Patterson AJ, et al. Thrombin activatable fibrinolysis inhibitor, a potential regulator of vascular inflammation. The Journal of Biological Chemistry. 2003;**278**:51059-51067. DOI: 10.1074/jbc.M306977200

[7] Zhou Q, Zhao L, Shao Z, Declerck P, Leung LLK, Morser J. Both plasma basic carboxypeptidases, carboxypeptidase B2 and carboxypeptidase N, regulate vascular leakage activity in mice. Journal of Thrombosis and Haemostasis: JTH. 2022;**20**:238-244. DOI: 10.1111/jth.15551

[8] Schieffer E, Schieffer B. The race for ACE: Targeting angiotensin-converting enzymes (ACE) in SARS-CoV-2 infection. Journal of the Renin-Angiotensin-Aldosterone System. 2022;**2022**:2549063. DOI: 10.1155/2022/2549063

[9] Tabassum A, Iqbal MS, Sultan S, Alhuthali RA, Alshubaili DI, Sayyam RS, et al. Dysregulated bradykinin: Mystery in the pathogenesis of COVID-19. Mediators of Inflammation. 2022;**2022**:7423537. DOI: 10.1155/2022/7423537

[10] Carvalho PRd, Sirois P, Fernandes PD. The role of kallikrein-kinin and renin-angiotensin systems in COVID-19 infection. Peptides. 2021;**135**:170428. DOI: 10.1016/j.peptides.2020.170428

[11] Lawal IO, Kgatle MM, Mokoala K, Farate A, Sathekge MM. Cardiovascular disturbances in COVID-19: An updated review of the pathophysiology and clinical evidence of cardiovascular damage induced by SARS-CoV-2. BMC Cardiovascular Disorders. 2022;**22**:93. DOI: 10.1186/s12872-022-02534-8

[12] Leung LLK, Morser J. Carboxypeptidase B2 and carboxypeptidase N in the crosstalk between coagulation, thrombosis, inflammation, and innate immunity. Journal of Thrombosis and Haemostasis: JTH. 2018;**16**(8):1474-1486. DOI: 10.1111/jth.14199

[13] Miszta A, Huskens D, Donkervoort D, Roberts MJM, Wolberg AS, Laat B. de.

Assessing plasmin generation in health and disease. International Journal of Molecular Sciences. 2021;**22**:2758-2774. DOI:10.3390/ijms22052758

[14] Elbasan O, Bayram F, Yazan CD, Apaydın T, Dashdamirova S, Polat H, et al. Angiotensin-converting enzyme (ACE) level, but not ACE gene polymorphism, is associated with prognosis of COVID-19 infection: Implications for diabetes and hypertension. PLoS One. 2023;**18**:e0288338. DOI: 10.1371/journal.pone.0288338

[15] Zobel CM, Kuhn H, Schreiner M, Wenzel W, Wendtland J, Goekeri C, et al. Impact of ACE I gene insertion/deletion, A-240T polymorphisms and the renin-angiotensin-aldosterone system on COVID-19 disease. Virology Journal. 2024;**21**:15. DOI: 10.1186/s12985-023-02283-w

[16] Alfaro E, Díaz-García E, García-Tovar S, Zamarrón E, Mangas A, Galera R, et al. Impaired Kallikrein-Kinin system in COVID-19 patient's severity. Frontiers in Immunology. 2022;**13**:909342. DOI: 10.3389/fimmu.2022.909342

[17] Bayer M, König S. A vote for robustness: Monitoring serum enzyme activity by thin-layer chromatography of dabsylated bradykinin products. Journal of Pharmaceutical and Biomedical Analysis. 2017;**143**:199-203. DOI: 10.1016/j.jpba.2017.06.007

[18] König S, Bayer M, Dimova V, Herrnberger M, Escolano-Lozano F, Bednarik J, et al. The serum protease network-one key to understand complex regional pain syndrome pathophysiology. Pain. 2019;**160**:1402-1409. DOI: 10.1097/j.pain.0000000000001503

[19] König S, Steinebrey N, Herrnberger M, Escolano-Lozano F, Schlereth T, Rebhorn C, et al. Reduced serum protease activity in complex regional pain syndrome: The impact of angiotensin-converting enzyme and carboxypeptidases. Journal of Pharmaceutical and Biomedical Analysis. 2021;**205**:114307. DOI: 10.1016/j.jpba.2021.114307

[20] Tepasse P-R, Vollenberg R, Steinebrey N, König S. High angiotensin-converting enzyme and low carboxypeptidase N serum activity correlate with disease severity in COVID-19 patients. Journal of Personalized Medicine. 2022;**12**:406. DOI: 10.3390/jpm12030406

[21] Tepasse P-R, Vollenberg R, Steinebrey N, König S. The dysregulation of the renin-angiotensin system in COVID-19 studied by serum proteomics: Angiotensinogen increases with disease severity. Molecules. 2022;**27**:2495. DOI: 10.3390/molecules27082495

[22] König S, Vollenberg R, Tepasse P-R. The renin-angiotensin system in COVID-19: Can long COVID be predicted? Life. 2023;**13**:1462. DOI: 10.3390/life13071462

[23] Abiola J, Berg AM, Aiyelaagbe O, Adeyi A, König S. Dabsylated bradykinin is cleaved by snake venom proteases from Echis ocellatus. Biomedicine. 2024;**12**:1027. DOI: 10.3390/biomedicines12051027

[24] Krasowski MD. Educational case: Hemolysis and Lipemia interference with laboratory testing. Academic Pathology. 2019;**6**:2374289519888754. DOI: 10.1177/2374289519888754

[25] Saenger JA, Atamaniuk J, Gaggl M, Asenbaum J, Huber FA, Grieb A, et al. Increased hemolysis rate in plasma tubes after implementation of a fully automated sample delivery and acceptance system. Journal

of Laboratoriums Medizin. 2023:**47**(2):63-68

[26] Wan Azman WN, Omar J, Koon TS, Tuan Ismail TS. Hemolyzed specimens: Major challenge for identifying and rejecting specimens in clinical laboratories. Oman Medical Journal. 2019;**34**:94-98. DOI: 10.5001/omj.2019.19

[27] Hernaningsih Y, Akualing JS. The effects of hemolysis on plasma prothrombin time and activated partial thromboplastin time tests using photo-optical method. Medicine. 2017;**96**:e7976. DOI: 10.1097/MD.0000000000007976

[28] Koseoglu M, Hur A, Atay A, Cuhadar S. Effects of hemolysis interferences on routine biochemistry parameters. Biochemia Medica. 2011;**21**:79-85. DOI: 10.11613/bm.2011.015

[29] Roman Y, Bomsel-Demontoy M-C, Levrier J, Chaste-Duvernoy D, Jalme MS. Effect of hemolysis on plasma protein levels and plasma electrophoresis in birds. Journal of Wildlife Diseases. 2009;**45**:73-80. DOI: 10.7589/0090-3558-45.1.73

[30] El-Khoury JM, Bunch DR, Wang S. Is the effect of hemolysis on plasma ammonia measurement overrated? Archives of Pathology and Laboratory Medicine. 2012;**136**:471-472. DOI: 10.5858/arpa.2011-0445-LE

[31] American Association of Zoo Veterinarians Conference 1997. VIN.com; Houston, TX. Oct 2020:26-30

[32] Marques-Garcia F, Jung DHH, Pérez SE. Impact of individualized hemolysis management based on biological variation cut-offs in a clinical laboratory. Annals of Laboratory Medicine. 2022;**42**:169-177. DOI: 10.3343/alm.2022.42.2.169

[33] Cdc. Reference Tool to Determine Hemolysis Status. Available from: https://www.cdc.gov/vector-borne-diseases/php/laboratories/reference-tool-for-hemolysis-status.html [Accessed: May 22, 2024].

[34] Ni J, Zhu W, Wang Y, Wei X, Li J, Peng L, et al. A reference chart for clinical biochemical tests of hemolyzed serum samples. Journal of Clinical Laboratory Analysis. 2021;**35**:e23561. DOI: 10.1002/jcla.23561

[35] Lippi G, Cadamuro J. Visual assessment of sample quality: Quo usque tandem? Clinical Chemistry and Laboratory Medicine (CCLM). 2018;**56**:513-515. DOI: 10.1515/cclm-2017-0867

[36] Gislefoss RE, Berge U, Lauritzen M, Langseth H, Wojewodzic MW. A simple and cost-effective method for measuring hemolysis in biobank serum specimens. Biopreservation and Biobanking. 2021;**19**:525-530. DOI: 10.1089/bio.2021.0037

[37] Ishiguro A, Nishioka M, Morishige A, Yoneshiro M, Shinkawa K, Fujinaga A, et al. Determination of the optimal wavelength of the hemolysis index measurement. Journal of Clinical Medicine. 2023;**12**:5864. DOI: 10.3390/jcm12185864

[38] Larrán B, López-Alonso M, Miranda M, Pereira V, Rigueira L, Suárez ML, et al. Measuring haemolysis in cattle serum by direct UV-VIS and RGB digital image-based methods. Scientific Reports. 2022;**12**:13523. DOI: 10.1038/s41598-022-17842-4

[39] Yang C, Li D, Sun D, Zhang S, Zhang P, Xiong Y, et al. A deep learning-based system for assessment of serum quality using sample images. Clinica Chimica Acta. 2022;**531**:254-260. DOI: 10.1016/j.cca.2022.04.010

[40] Searfoss R, Shah P, Ofori-Mensa K, Bussberg V, Tolstikov V, Greenwood B, et al. Impact of hemolysis on multi-OMIC pancreatic biomarker discovery to derisk biomarker development in precision medicine studies. Scientific Reports. 2022;**12**:1186. DOI: 10.1038/s41598-022-05152-8

[41] König S, Schork K, Eisenacher M. Observations from the proteomics bench. Proteomes. 2024;**12**:6. DOI: 10.3390/proteomes12010006

[42] Schreiber U, Engl C, Bayer M, König S. Neuropeptide reporter assay for serum, capillary blood and blood cards. MethodsX. 2020;**7**:100985. DOI: 10.1016/j.mex.2020.100985

[43] Schreiber U, Bayer M, König S. Validation data for the use of bradykinin and substance P protease activity assays with capillary blood and blood cards. Data in Brief. 2020;**28**:104873. DOI: 10.1016/j.dib.2019.104873

Chapter 5

Subclinical Hypercortisolism

Gilson de Abreu Viza Junior

Abstract

Acid-base homeostasis is fundamental for the maintenance of life. Subclinical hypercortisolism (HS) is an entity that is difficult to diagnose as it does not present a noticeable symptomatological picture without advanced resources for clinical practice. The objective of this chapter is to discuss the importance of recognizing this entity and establishing differential diagnosis. Characterization of those elements is the way for provide a good clinical practice and avoid mistakes. The cortisol and other glucocorticoids which have the ability to stimulate gluconeogenesis are the target of his study. An up-to-date approach is proposed. This is a narrative review carried out between 1993 and 2024. The following databases were used: DOAJ Directory of Open Access Journals; PubMed, PubMed(Medline).

Keywords: hypercortisolism, hyperglycemia, diabetic neuropathy, aldosterone, hypertension, infection, cellular adaptation to stress

1. Introduction

The interpretation of acid-base disorders is considered an essential skill for all physicians, regardless of their training or specialty. The rapid recognition of an acid-base disorder can save lives, but its diagnosis can be challenging. Correct identification of the presence of acid-base disorders depends on understanding the pathophysiological mechanisms that generate them, combined with a systematic interpretation that involves history and physical examination data, determination of the primary disorder, estimation of compensatory responses, assessment of coexisting metabolic distress and calculation of the osmolar gap in metabolic acidosis with increased anion-gap (AG) [1]. This chapter places special emphasis on increased cortisol concentration and hypercortisolism.

Hypercortisolism presents a very common differential diagnosis in public health, which is diabetes mellitus (DM), which initially manifests itself through hyperglycemia, measured through the collection of a morning blood sample. Subclinical hypercortisolism (HS) is an entity that is difficult to diagnose as it does not present a noticeable symptomatological picture without advanced resources for clinical practice. It is a disease characterized by increased blood serum levels of cortisol, a corticosteroid hormone measured through blood or saliva samples.

The high amount of cortisol in the bloodstream could be misunderstood by high levels of glucose, sepsis and any hyperosmolar particle that is able to travel in the blood, an effect known as cross-reaction. That is why we need enhanced resources to distinguish the difference between them, for example, high levels of glucose lead to *diabetes mellitus* and high levels of bacteria in the blood samples (bacteremia) lead to sepsis. *Hypercortisolism*, on the other hand, is a high level of *cortisol*, a corticosteroid hormone produced by the cortex of adrenal.

2. Hypercortisolism

There are three distinct clinical hyperadrenal syndromes (1) *Cushing's syndrome*, characterized by an excess of cortisol, (2) *hyperaldosteronism* and (3) *adrenogenital* or *virilizing syndrome*. *Cushing syndrome*, is a common manifestation of *hypercortisolism*, caused by any condition that produces an increase in glucocorticoid levels [2].

In clinical practice, the vast majority of cases of Cushing's syndrome result from the administration of exogenous (iatrogenic) glucocorticoids. The remaining cases are endogenous, and the three most common etiological disorders are:

1. Primary hypothalamic-pituitary diseases associated with ACTH hypersecretion.
2. Ectopic ACTH secretion by nonpituitary neoplasms.
3. Primary adrenocortical neoplasms (adenoma or carcinoma) and, rarely, primary cortical hyperplasia [2].

The mineralocorticoids synthesize in the adrenal cortex, the most important being aldosterone, which is generated in the zona glomerulosa; it occurs in response to activation of the renin-angiotensin system or can be released primarily by the autonomous produce, with resultant suppression of the renin-angiotensin system and decreased plasma renin activity [2].

The regulation of aldosterone secretion is so deeply intertwined with the regulation of extracellular fluid electrolyte concentrations, extracellular fluid volume, blood volume, blood pressure and many special aspects of renal function that it is difficult to discuss it independently of all these factors [3].

Four factors are identified to play essential roles in the regulation of aldosterone. In likely order of importance, these factors are:

1. High concentrations of potassium ions in the extracellular fluid greatly increase aldosterone secretion.
2. Elevated activity of the renin-angiotensin system (increased levels of angiotensin II) also significantly increases aldosterone secretion.
3. Increasing sodium ion concentrations in the extracellular fluid only slightly reduces aldosterone secretion.
4. ACTH formed by the anterior pituitary is necessary for aldosterone secretion but has a weak effect on controlling the rate of secretion [3].

3. The cortisol

The most widely known metabolic effect of cortisol and other glucocorticoids is their ability to stimulate gluconeogenesis (the formation of carbohydrates from proteins and some other substances) by the liver, the activity of which is often increased six- to tenfold.

This is mainly due to two effects of cortisol:

1. *Cortisol enhances the enzymes required for the concentration of amino acids into glucose by liver cells*. This is due to the cause of glucocorticoids on the activation of transcription of DNA in the nuclei of liver cells, action similar to that of aldosterone in renal tubular cells, with formation of messenger RNAs that in turn generate the set of enzymes necessary for gluconeogenesis.

2. *Cortisol causes the mobilization of amino acids from extrahepatic tissues, mainly from muscle.* As a result, more amino acids are made available in the plasma to enter the process of gluconeogenesis by the liver and thus promote the formation of glucose [3].

One effect of increased gluconeogenesis is an increase in glycogen stores in liver cells. This effect of cortisol allows other glycolytic hormones, such as epinephrine and glucagon, to mobilize glucose at times of need, such as between meals [3]. A contrast finding from abdominal ultrasound imaging confirms that this liver sickness is hepatic steatosis.

Cortisol also moderately reduces the rate at which glucose is utilized by most cells in the body. Although the cause of this decrease is unknown, most physiologists think that cortisol directly decreases the rate at which glucose is utilized at some point between its entry into cells and its final degradation. One suggested mechanism is based on the observation that glucocorticoids reduce the oxidation of nicotinamide adenine dinucleotide (NADH) to form NAD+. Since NADH oxidation is necessary to enable glycolysis, this effect may be responsible for the negative feedback utilization of glucose by cells [3]. The cortisol hormone diagram (**Figure 1**) exemplifies the effects of this hormone on the body.

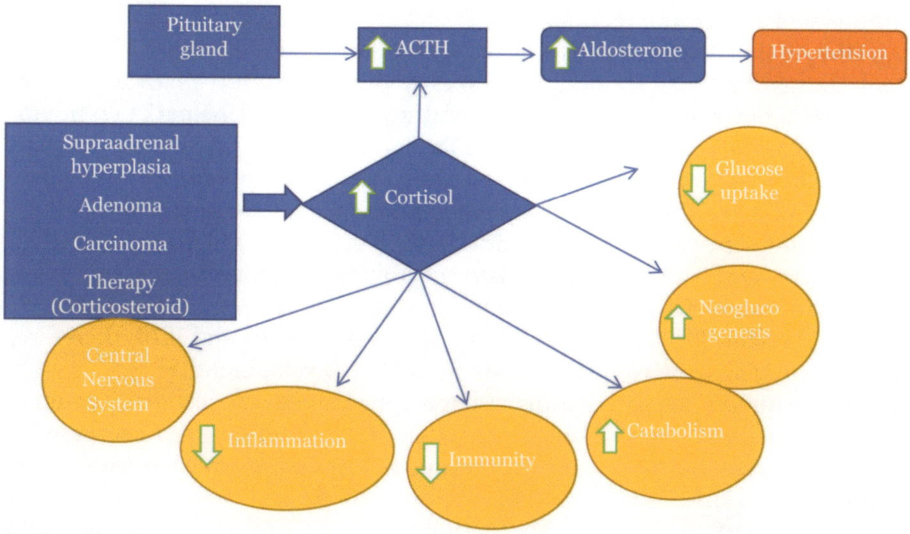

Figure 1.
Cortisol hormone diagram.

Both the elevated rate of gluconeogenesis and the moderate reduction in the rate at which glucose is utilized by cells cause an elevation in blood glucose concentration. This elevation, in turn, stimulates insulin secretion. Higher plasma insulin levels, however, are not as effective in maintaining plasma glucose as they are under normal conditions. For reasons that are not fully understood, high glucocorticoid levels reduce the sensitivity of many tissues, especially skeletal muscle and adipose tissue, to the stimulatory effects of insulin on glucose adaptation and utilization. One possible explanation is that high fatty acid levels, caused by the effect of glucocorticoids on mobilizing lipids from fat stores, may impair the actions of insulin in tissues. Thus, excess glucocorticoid secretion can produce disturbances in carbohydrate metabolism that are very similar to those found in patients with excessive levels of growth hormone [3]. This produces an increase in the amount of accumulated mass in the body which can be translated as obesity.

The rise in blood glucose concentration is sometimes so great (50% or more above normal) that the condition is called adrenal diabetes. Insulin administration reduces blood glucose concentration only moderately in adrenal diabetes—much less than in pancreatic diabetes—because the tissues are resistant to the effects of insulin [3]. A usual symptom resulting from this elevation of blood glucose is the excretion of glucose in the urine and glycosuria.

Childhood obesity is defined as a body mass index (BMI) above the 97th percentile, adjusted for sex and age. It is considered a multisystemic condition associated with enhanced release and activation of pro-inflammatory cells and cytokines, resulting in dysregulation of the immune system. Furthermore, obesity is associated with dysfunctions of the main endocrine and metabolic pathways, increasing the risk of other morbidities, such as those related to metabolic syndrome (hypertension, diabetes and dyslipidemia), as well as ailment in other systems, such as the integumentary system [4].

Obesity, recognized as a chronic inflammatory disease, plays a significant role in the development of several dermatological conditions. Chronic low-grade inflammation, together with activation of the immune system, maybe the shared pathological basis of obesity-associated skin disorders [4]. Skin fragmentation evolves into a cutaneous sign known as striae.

An allergic skin disease well associated with obesity, described in the literature, is atopic dermatitis (AD), formerly known as atopic eczema. It is characterized as a chronic inflammatory illness associated with an increase in T helper2 (Th2) lymphocytes. Both AD and obesity, or other inflammatory conditions such as diabetes mellitus, present a similar overproduction of cytokines and inflammatory mediators, suggesting a possible shared causal association between these diseases [4].

A surprising aspect of Th17 differentiation is that TGF-β, which is produced by many cell types and is an anti-inflammatory cytokine, promotes the development of pro-inflammatory Th17 cells when other mediators of inflammation, such as IL-6 or IL-1, are present. Th17 differentiation is inhibited by IFN-γ and IL-4; therefore, strong Th1 and Th2 responses tend to suppress Th17 development [5].

Since neutrophils are a predominant defense mechanism against many common bacteria and fungi, Th17 cells play an important role in defending against these infections. Th17 cells combat microbes by recruiting leukocytes, mainly neutrophils, to sites of infection [5].

Th17 cells contribute to the pathogenesis of many inflammatory diseases. The Th17 response has been associated with psoriasis, inflammatory bowel disease, rheumatoid arthritis and multiple sclerosis. Agents that block the development or function of

Th17 cells are in clinical trials for several of these diseases and are approved for the treatment of psoriasis. These antagonists are not effective in inflammatory bowel disease and perhaps also in rheumatoid arthritis, so the role of Th17 cells in these diseases is unclear. Both Th1 and Th17 cells may be present in lesions in several inflammatory diseases, and both may contribute to the development and propagation of these disorders [5].

The frequency with which the nervous system is affected by diabetes was undoubtedly responsible for the initial idea that diabetes was caused by a disease of the nervous system. It was not until 1864 that the opposite was initially recognized [6].

In the literature on diabetic neuropathy, a distinction has been made between "peripheral" and "autonomic" neuropathy, without recognizing that the word "peripheral" refers to the peripheral nervous system and not to the distribution of the neuropathy. The peripheral nervous system has both somatic and autonomic components [6].

Although the autonomic nervous system is traditionally referred to as an efferent system, for innervation of visceral smooth muscle, it is important to include the visceral afferent fibers that accompany it. Therefore, diabetic autonomic neuropathy encompasses multiple disturbances of the motor, sensory and reflex functions, particularly affecting the cardiovascular, gastrointestinal and urogenital systems. In addition, there is also damage to the sudomotor and vasomotor thermoregulatory mechanisms, the reflex pupillary function and the endocrine control mechanisms [6]. Central nervous system involvement can be recognized by symptoms of depression, psychosis and mood changes.

There is poor literature on pathological studies of the vagus nerve in patients known to have chronic autonomic diabetic neuropathy. Morphological studies of the vagus nerve have mostly been conducted in its abdominal segment, demonstrating a severe decrease in the density of unmyelinated fibers, with the "surviving" axons being of small diameter [6].

Endogenous Cushing's syndrome (CS) is an endocrine pathology rare with an approximate incidence of 0.2 to 5 cases per million inhabitants per year. Up to 25% are independent of adrenocorticotropin (ACTH), and the remaining 75% are dependent on the same, 70% being of pituitary origin, known as Cushing's disease (CD). Only 5% are often associated with an ectopic origin of ACTH production, frequently in the setting of a neuroendocrine tumor. The Ectopic Cushing's syndrome (ECS) poses a diagnostic challenge and has an elevated morbidity and mortality rate due to its common association with comorbidities, delays in diagnosis and treatment that lead to an increase in the risk of thromboembolism pulmonary, sepsis, opportunistic or disseminated parasitic infection, heart failure, gastrointestinal bleeding, psychosis acute, progressive, debilitating myopathy, hypokalemia uncontrolled, hypertension and/or hyperglycemia. There is no clear definition of severe hypercortisolism; however, biochemical findings, such as random serum cortisol greater than 40 Ug/dL, elevation of urinary free cortisol of 24 hours above five times the upper limit of normal and/or severe hypokalemia, are often related to clinical presentations of severe CS [7].

Chronicity and cortisol levels will determine the severity of clinical appearance. Changes are usually described phenotypic such as plethora, full moon face, abdominal stretch marks violet, buffalo hump, central obesity, muscle weakness proximal; clinical manifestations that are not specific to a particular type of CS and are not present in all patients. Hypertension arterial and diabetes mellitus, generally difficult to control, are often associated with this entity. In the case pointed out, the patient had no usual phenotypic demonstrations; he had a diagnosis of recent diabetes and hypertension associated with hypokalemia, severe, persistent and difficult to manage. There has been recorded a frequency association between electrolyte disturbances and acid-base balance with hypokalemia and metabolic alkalosis with ECS, so in those cases where a document does not provide apparent cause or in those that do not respond adequately when handling standard it is indicated to evaluate cortisol levels as part of the differential diagnosis; which may be present up to 70% of cases of Cushing's syndrome and less than 10% of Cushing's disease (CD) [7].

Measurements of salivary cortisol at night, 24-hour urine-free cortisol excretion, or a 1-mg dexamethasone suppression test at night are essential to identify hypercortisolism. In our case, we found a high 24-hour urinary cortisol level, paradoxical suppression of serum cortisol after oral dexamethasone, and elevated ACTH, thus establishing the presence of severe ACTH-dependent hypercortisolism. In CD, we basically find an inadequate cortisol response to the post-dexamethasone brake, which confirms the excess in its production, but in ectopic causes, this response can become paradoxical with higher cortisol values after the brake because ACTH production is higher when compared to that derived from corticotropic pituitary tumors. A test can be performed with elevated doses of dexamethasone based on the fact that ACTH secretion by pituitary adenomas is only relatively resistant to the negative feedback regulation exerted by glucocorticoids. On the other hand, most nonpituitary tumors associated with ectopic ACTH secretion are completely resistant to this feedback inhibition. It should also be stated that this test is not very specific, since up to 20% of patients with CD do not respond; so, it is necessary to document with imaging the pituitary or extrapituitary cause of ACTH production [7].

With the diagnosis of ACTH-dependent CS, the first cause to be ruled out is the presence of a pituitary adenoma. The image of choice is magnetic resonance imaging of the sella turcica and in certain cases ACTH levels can be measured in the inferior petrosal venous sinuses. If the presence of a pituitary adenoma is ruled out, the location of an ACTH-producing tumor or neuroendocrine tumor (NET) should be evaluated; often are pulmonary; small cell lung carcinoma, lung carcinoid tumor or thymic carcinoid tumors (5–42%). The location of the ACTH-secreting tumor is difficult, so different imaging techniques have been studied to enhance diagnosis. Studies can be improved with abdominal tomography, since they also occur in pancreatic tumors (7.5–25%), pheochromocytomas (2.5–25%), and much less frequently in the gastrointestinal tract, prostate and medullary thyroid cancer (2–8%). In our case, bilateral adrenal hyperplasia and a pulmonary nodule at the right paracardiac level were registered. There are no imaging studies that are the gold standard to show all neuroendocrine tumors, and up to 10 to 20% of patients may remain without identifying their source. The majority of tumors related to ectopic ACTH secretion are neuroendocrine and have an overexpression of the somatostatin receptor (70–90% of cases). For positron emission tomography (PET scan) using gallium 68 or 18 fluorodeoxyglucose, sensitivity is high for the diagnosis of bronchial carcinoids. Approximately 20% of ACTH-dependent SCs identified by PET scan are from a pulmonary source [7].

4. Conclusions

The main disease addressed in this narrative can be properly characterized and differentiated from other clinical entities that are important in clinical practice. The symptoms elucidated in this study encompass several organic systems that translate as pain in the musculoskeletal system, osmotic diuresis in the renal system, weight gain in the endocrine system, striae in the integumentary system, infections that can be localized or even generalized, depression, psychosis and mood changes in the central nervous system. Subclinical hypercortisolism (SH), despite being a milder form of the disease, was properly characterized in this study based on its pathophysiology. All of this was differentiated from what occurs in other comorbidities, the main one being *diabetes mellitus*.

The suspected diagnosis was discussed through advanced complementary examinations collected from biological samples that brought markers and antigens intrinsic to each process of establishing the disease. In hypercortisolism, the presence of cortisol is decisive for diagnostic confirmation, so the clinical reasoning developed throughout the study that characterizes this disease must be perfect.

The exclusion of diabetes mellitus must be a goal of clinical practice, since this comorbidity presents points of intersection that confuse clinical reasoning for other diseases due to its wide variety of alterations that occur at the biochemical level. Other symptoms that characterize it include polydipsia, polyphagia, obesity, stroke, thrombosis, atheromatosis and neuropathic pain. Knowledge of this clinical picture facilitates the beginning of the dialog between the two clinical entities addressed in this study, in order to establish a limit that separates them.

With the acquired and updated knowledge of the two diseases, it becomes possible to establish this limit between the two in clinical practice.

Acknowledgements

To God, my family and my advisor.
Funding resources were denied by the filiation institution.

Conflict of interest

The authors declare no conflict of interest.

Notes/acknowledgements/other declarations

I would like to thank my institution, Universidade Federal do Tocantins, which provided access to all databases used.

Author details

Gilson de Abreu Viza Junior
Universidade Federal do Tocantins, Palmas, Brasil

*Address all correspondence to: gilsonjrdr@hotmail.com

References

[1] Martins HS. Medicina de emergência: revisão rápida. Barueri, SP: Manole; 2016

[2] Kumar V, Abbas AK, Fausto N, Mitchell RN. Robbins Basic Pathology. 9. ed. Philadelphia: Saunders-Elsevier; 2013

[3] Guyton AC. In: Guyton AC, Hall JE, de Alencar Martins B, et al., editors. 1919-2003 Textbook of Medical Physiology. 4th ed. Rio de Janeiro: Elsevier; 2006

[4] Martins JÁE, de Nogueira AKA, de Vasconcelos CBS, Rodríguez VC, da Costa RSL. Manifestações dermatológicas em crianças com obesidade: Uma revisão integrativa de literatura. Revista Foco [S. l.]. 2024;**17**(4):e4762. DOI: 10.54751/revistafoco.v17n4-080. Available from: https://ojs.focopublicacoes.com.br/foco/article/view/4762

[5] Abbas AK, Pillai S, Lichtman AH. Immunology: Cellular and Molecular. 9th ed. Rio De Janeiro: Editora Elsevier Ltda; 2019

[6] Sato KL, Migliaccio V, Carmo JM, Oliveti MCDBB, Ferreira RS, Fazan VPS. Diabetes as a model of autonomic neuropathy. Medicina (Ribeirão Preto). 2006;**39**(1):28-38

[7] Cione LA, Colletti LF. Severe hypercortisolism and recurrent hypokalemia. Arquivos Médicos e Patológicos. 2022;**39**(2):236-244. DOI: 10.35663/amp.2022.392.2363